AF709316

Interviewing the Patient

GEORGE L. ENGEL, M.D.

Professor of Psychiatry and Professor of Medicine, The University of Rochester School of Medicine and Dentistry

WILLIAM L. MORGAN, Jr., M.D.

Professor of Medicine, The University of Rochester School of Medicine and Dentistry

W. B. Saunders Company Ltd *London • Philadelphia • Toronto*

W. B. Saunders Company: West Washington Square
Philadelphia, Pa. 19105

1 St. Anne's Road
Eastbourne, East Sussex BN21 3UN, England

833 Oxford Street
Toronto, M8Z 5T9, Canada

Interviewing the Patient **ISBN 0-7216-3393-5**

© 1973 by W. B. Saunders Company Ltd. Adapted from: *The Clinical Approach to the Patient,* © 1969 by W. B. Saunders Company. Copyright under the International Copyright Union. All rights reserved. This book is protected by copyright. No part of it may be reproduced, stored in a retrieval system, or transmitted in any form or by any means, electronic, mechanical, photocopying, recording or otherwise, without written permission from the publisher. Library of Congress catalog card number 73-81834.

Made in the United States of America.
Press of W. B. Saunders Company.

Print No.: 9 8 7 6 5 4 3 2

Dedicated to
Our Students

Contents

Introduction

The decision to make available as a separate volume the material on interviewing from *The Clinical Approach to the Patient* reflects a demand by some for a smaller and less expensive volume devoted to the area most neglected in other texts. We have acceded reluctantly for we value the essential unity of the book as a whole and urge strongly that medical students in particular use the full text. This version contains unchanged the first three chapters and the verbatim interview in the Appendix.

We are also taking this opportunity to elaborate on the functions of the interview in medical practice and to offer some suggestions to teachers undertaking this important discipline.

The Role of the Interview in Medical Practice

The ability to interview patients skillfully represents far more than merely a technique to collect clinical data, important as that may be. It is in fact the keystone of the physician's clinical skills and the basis for effective communication between him and his patient. Without the ability to interview skillfully, the physician cannot fully comprehend his patient's needs, nor can his patient grasp or comply with his directions and expectations. Virtually indispensable for physician–patient interaction, the well-conducted interview truly may be regarded as the most powerful, the most sensitive, and the most versatile instrument available to the physician. Indeed, one can hardly think of any clinical situation in which a verbal exchange is not required for effective care and treatment. Let the physician who doubts this premise recall his sense of impotence when confronted with a patient with whom he cannot speak and about whom no other source of information is available.

1) The interview is the medium through which a relationship is initiated, developed, and sustained, often between two strangers who must in short order establish the foundations upon which one seeks help from the other. This complementarity of the need for help on the part of the patient and the wish and capability to help on the part of the physician facilitates the initiation of the interview and the interpersonal interaction. What transpires verbally and nonverbally between patient and physician in the very first minutes of this encounter may profoundly influence not only the subsequent course of the interview but also the very nature of the relationship that ultimately evolves.

2) Through the process of the interview both the physician and the patient identify what is required for each to communicate effectively with the other. The patient, to enlist help from the physician, must quickly ascertain what kind of information and behavior are expected from him in order for the physician to provide that help. The physician in turn must familiarize himself with the patient's style of communication while clarifying for the patient what he needs to fulfill his responsibility to help. The physician encourages the patient to formulate his problems and concerns in his own words and takes careful note not only of the information given, but also of emphases, mannerisms, and other nonverbal behavior. Once he has become familiar with the patient's particular style of communicating he can then proceed by nods, gestures, comments or questions to indicate the particular areas of information that are most important to elaborate. The mutual understanding of each other's modes of communication so achieved is indispensable for obtaining reliable data and assuring subsequent compliance by the patient with the physician's instructions.

3) The interview defines the respective roles and obligations of physician and patient. This is a subtle process of negotiation that establishes the conditions under which the physician will accept responsibility for the patient and the patient will agree to entrust himself to the care of the physician. From the very beginning of the interview direct or subtle messages convey such information, whether a smile or a frown, an invitation or an order, a fearful question or an angry demand. A successful interview will be marked by the physician having conveyed to the patient the feeling that he cares while the patient in turn feels and communicates trust.

4) The best known objective of the interview is *data collection.* This includes eliciting the information necessary (a) to identify and define the nature of the patient's problems, (b) to delineate disease processes, (c) to characterize the patient as a person, (d) to define

his current and past life circumstances, and (e) to establish his biological, psychological and social strengths and resources as well as his weaknesses and deficiencies. Reliability and completeness of the interview are very much dependent upon the physician's success in first establishing a relationship, achieving fluent communication, and defining roles and obligations.

5) The interview is also a system for *data processing*. Far from being a simple structured activity in which a defined series of questions yield specific answers, the successive responses of both patient and physician are based on the interpretations by each of what has just transpired. For the physician the task is to make sense of what the patient is reporting. This is an interpretive process which ultimately involves reformulation of the patient's verbal report into various frames of reference relevant to concepts of health and illness. As he listens to his patient, the physician attempts in his own mind to order the information and to assign meaning, a process which involves continuous scanning of his own experience and knowledge for points of familiarity and congruence. This in essence constitutes a process of analysis and synthesis in the course of which the physician repeatedly constructs and tests hypotheses through further and directed inquiry of the patient until corroborating or refuting information emerges.

Clearly then the interview is an active, dynamic process, the effectiveness of which very much depends upon the physician's knowledge and experience as well as on his ability continuously to organize the information, to recognize its meaning, to test its significance, and yet remain open and receptive to that which resists interpretation. Central to the effectiveness of this process is not only the physician's knowledge but also his skill in influencing the patient to provide unbiased information.

6) In the course of the interview information emerges about the current and past personal, family, social and economic circumstances of the patient as well as about his previous experiences with illness and with health care. These provide the background to guide the physician as to how best to communicate his judgments and recommendations to the patient and family, to engage them effectively in their subsequent study, care and treatment, and to achieve their cooperation. The important responsibility of the physician to instruct patients in the requirements for their own care begins with the establishment of a trusting relationship and is facilitated by an accurate assessment of the emotional and intellectual capabilities of the patient and his family at various phases of the illness.

7) And finally through the interview and the other verbal interchanges between patient and physician a psychological contract emerges which defines the mutually acceptable conditions for continuing care. This has both long and short-term implications which are crucial to whether or not the patient thereafter thinks of the physician as "my doctor" and the physician thinks of the patient as "my patient". This expresses a deep and often lasting bond marked ideally by mutual trust, confidence and sense of responsibility which gives assurance that help can be solicited and care will be provided whenever the need may arise.

Some Principles Underlying Teaching Interviewing

Seen in its full scope, learning how to interview should enjoy the status of a major discipline in the education of the physician. This is clearly not so today. In most schools only the data collection function is recognized, the task being conceived as "history taking" for which no instruction or supervision is deemed necessary beyond the student learning the divisions of the written history and what questions to direct to the patient. In only a few schools are students ever supervised while interviewing patients and this occurs usually only once or twice early in their careers. Even more critical is the fact that few faculty have devoted effort to mastering either interviewing or to learning how to teach this skill Fewer still have ever had their own interviewing subjected to audit. Hence, the task of improving interviewing instruction is formidable. We hope the few comments here will serve to arouse interest in some of the approaches that may be utilized to teach interviewing skills to young physicians. Fortunately, the ready accessibility of audio and video recording equipment in most schools now provides a teaching resource especially useful for monitoring student performance.

An important question is how early in medical school should interview instruction be initiated? The student can learn a good deal early on by observing skillful interviewers work with patients. But his own efforts at interviewing are likely to be seriously hampered as long as he does not yet "feel" like a doctor and is deficient in the basic science and clinical knowledge required to understand and process the information provided by the patient. These deficiencies by no means preclude the student learning a good deal *about* interviewing early in medical school, but they do limit seriously his acquisition of the skills of interviewing required for the physician's task. Therefore in planning instruction it is necessary to identify what kind of exercises will be most useful early in the student training and which would better be delayed until the student has more background and experience. What follows conforms roughly to such a sequence and represents approaches to teaching interviewing that have been developed over many years at the University of Rochester.

1) *Learning to observe and report accurately.* Instruction may begin by having students observe how patients interact with the physician and how they relate their stories in an interview. Such interviews may be conducted even before large classes, especially if the auditorium is equipped with a one-way vision window and good sound equipment and the interview can be taped for replay before smaller groups. The latter setting, however, is indispensable if students are to become actively engaged. The student's initial task is to gain skill in organizing and reporting accurately the information elicited from the patient. Patients interviewed in a realistic clinical situation provide the best subjects for study while replay of video or audio tapes of the interview then allow the instructor to check the reliability of the reported observations. Students are introduced to the variability inherent in clinical work when they can observe several different physicians interview a variety of patients who demonstrate a range of problems. The instructor can facilitate organization of the interview material by encouraging students to think in terms of a crude classification of the problems that have been presented by the patient. At the outset interviews should be limited to not more than 15–20 minutes; any longer is simply overwhelming for beginning students who have difficulty in knowing what to be listening for. From the outset the instructor must impress upon students the need to be disciplined in the accuracy and completeness of their observation and reporting. First an observing student is asked to describe the patient, his physical appearance, dress, posture, expressions, activities, behavior, and interaction with the interviewing physician. Other students are invited to add to, correct or amend this description. Then another student is required to report his version of the patient's account of his illness and his life situation, and how he sees himself. Whether reported orally or in writing students learn much from comparing each other's accounts and discussing discrepancies. The instructor in turn monitors the accuracy of the reports, emphasizing in particular chronology, sequences, interrelationships and the importance of using the patient's own words or concepts, e.g. not to report "pain" when the patient described "pressure". Replay of the audio or video tape, which the student may do by himself, enables him to check on his own errors and to appreciate the principles imparted by the instructor.

2) *Learning how physician and patient communicate and relate with one another.* When the student has achieved some competence

in observing the patient's behavior and in accurately recording what the patient had reported, attention is shifted to the processes involved. The tapes of previously interviewed patients may be re-used to advantage for this purpose or new patients may be interviewed. The instructor points out and then students may be asked to note how the patient and the physician each express themselves. Attention is directed to the interaction between the two, particularly how the behavior of each, nonverbal as well as verbal, influences and determines the subsequent sequence of events. The influence on the course of the interview of open-ended versus direct questions, silence, facilitation, confrontation, and of reassurance and support may be pointed out. Half of the students may focus on the patient, the other half on the physician, and the ensuing discussion should bring together the two sets of observations. The interviewer himself may elaborate on the basis for his choice of questions and interventions at various points in the interview. This will inevitably introduce the student to the data processing aspect of the interview, a subject which assumes increasing importance with time. Other sessions may illustrate how both the physician and patient develop their relationships and define their roles with each other.

Demonstration exercises of this sort may be carried out before a large class but effective engagement of students is best accomplished in smaller groups, especially if audio or video tapes of the patient interview are available for more detailed examination. Students also learn much working by themselves in small groups with tape recordings if they are required to submit written reports.

3) *Learning to overcome the initial uneasiness of first contacts with patients.* The student's first encounters with patients cannot help but be artificial because he has not yet achieved a professional role with the patient. Even though more than willing to participate in the exercise, the patient does not have the same expectations and attitudes he would have with a physician or even with a more advanced student who is more involved in his care. Some patients even see their role more as helping the student than being helped. Because of this artificiality of the student's first interviews they must still be regarded as simulated medical interviews. Their main value is to help the student overcome his uneasiness and to experience being the interviewer rather than merely an observer. Such interviews should be brief, not more than 10–20 minutes, so as not to generate more data than the student can comfortably handle. It is imperative that the instructor also be present to observe the student's technique and to carry on further interviewing if it appears that an important principle or technique should be demonstrated. By having other students in the group as observers

and by playing back audio or video tape recordings of the interview the students have the opportunity to learn from each other's experiences.

These initial encounters can be effectively accomplished simply by an instructor taking a group of 6–8 students to the bedside or clinic. Since the interviews are brief several students can have an interview experience in a single session. In our own teaching we have also found no difficulty in having students conduct interviews behind the one-way screen before the whole class.

4) *Learning to interview in the evolving role of physician.* The exercises described so far may be considered only as preparatory to the main objective of learning how to interview as a physician. This requires that two criteria be fulfilled. First, the student must have a reasonable grasp of the languages and concepts of both the behavioral and the biological disciplines that are basic for an understanding of health, disease and the experience of illness. Second, he must be functioning as an active member of the group involved in the care of the patient. Only then can he personally experience the psychological and interpersonal aspects of the complementary relationship that develops between physician and patient and begin to cope with the essential task of interpreting the information from the patient.

Successful mastery of interviewing and of the patient-physician relationship in this context requires ongoing and continuing supervision throughout the student's clinical work. It is a serious error to assume that this can be successfully accomplished in a circumscribed block of time at the beginning of the student's clinical work and that no further follow-up is necessary. A student needs much experience and help to acquire the background with patients and with disease necessary for him to be able to subject the interview data to the analytic processes of clinical reasoning, clinical judgment, and clinical decision making.

For this phase of the instruction to be more effective the student should be assigned to a clinical unit where he is seen by patients as involved with the staff responsible for their care. At the same time this enables the student to begin to feel more at home in the clinical setting and to have house staff and faculty available as role models. He has the opportunity to become familiar with the ward structure and routine and to enjoy the experience of engaging for the first time in the work of a physician. At Rochester this is accomplished in a 12-week General Clerkship where there are no competing assignments and students are assigned fulltime to a clinical unit.[1]

---

[1]Morgan, W. L., Engel, G. L., and Luria, M. N.: The General Clerkship. A Course Designed to Teach the Clinical Approach to the Patient. J. Med. Educ. *47*:556–563, 1972.

Instruction begins with a series of relatively brief interviews with different patients conducted at the bedside which lengthen progressively in subsequent sessions until a complete history is secured. It is appropriate to devote the first exercise only to the first three steps of the interview, as outlined in the text, i.e. introducing oneself to the patient, putting the patient at ease, and establishing the major areas of complaint (See text). This may be accomplished in as little as 5 minutes in the context of the student being a new staff member becoming acquainted with the patients on the ward. In this manner a group of six students may in rapid succession see six to eight patients with an instructor and have their efforts immediately evaluated. Thereafter subsequent sessions with new patients may be expanded to 10, 20 and finally 40 minutes to an hour. In every instance each interview should progress through the steps given in the text. It is a mistake to assign students on one occasion to elicit the present illness and on another family health or personal and social history. These represent categories for recording the data and do not correspond with how information normally emerges in a well-conducted interview. Hence for each session the student is informed how much time he is expected to devote to interviewing, whether 10 minutes or an hour, and instructed to bring the interview to an end at that time without regard to completeness. Only as he achieves increasing facility in interviewing, which may not be for a year or more, is more attention paid to accomplishing a full interview in a briefer time. For the beginner an hour or even two hours of interviewing will be needed to complete the history.

For all exercises an instructor should be present to observe the student's interview which should also be tape recorded so that it can later be reviewed with the instructor. The rare student who is made uneasy by the presence of observers may be permitted to tape record his interview and then review and discuss the tape interview with an instructor. In general such exercises are best conducted with at least three, but not more than six, students present. Groups of this size allow for more effective and less charged peer interactions. It is good practice to begin with the interviewer evaluating his own performance, not omitting his feelings of ease or discomfort and his attitudes towards the patient. Then the observing students can contribute their opinions. Selected segments of the tape recording may be used to verify or reinforce points made by the discussants. It is good practice for the instructor to identify the good points of the student's technique as well as to point out errors.

There is no established number of supervised interviewing sessions that may be regarded as sufficient for this introductory period. It is doubtful that there can be too many, the limiting factor more likely being faculty and patient availability. More important is continuing supervision. This may best be accomplished by departing from the traditional case presentation method of bedside teaching and requiring the student to demonstrate his ability to interview and relate to the patient at the outset of the rounds. We recommend that before a patient is presented a student who does not know the patient conduct an interview for 10 to 15 minutes in the presence of the instructor and his fellow students. In this way the group are able not only to observe the student's interview skills but also are in position to subject the data so obtained to at least preliminary analysis which may be checked against what had already been learned about the patient by others. This approach to clinical teaching is described in more detail elsewhere.[2]

General appreciation of the importance of interviewing for medical practice is just beginning to develop among medical educators. In the future we can anticipate more scholarly studies of the nature of this important process as well as more imaginative and effective approaches to teaching.

---

[2]Engel, G. L.: Some Limitations of the Case Presentation Method for Clinical Teaching. An Alternative Approach. New Eng. J. Med. *284*:20–24, 1971.

Chapter 1

INTRODUCTION TO THE PATIENT

BEGINNING CLINICAL WORK

The education of the clinical student is conducted in a setting entirely different from the preclinical years. For the first time other human beings are the direct objects of study, and his work with them includes responsibility for their well-being. No longer can the student determine the conditions under which his material will be studied, as was the case in the physiology laboratory or the autopsy room. Clinical education is founded upon a unique human bond, the physician-patient relationship, without which the patient is unable or unwilling to share the information necessary for the student to understand and learn about disease.

The purpose of this book is to help the student undertake clinical responsibilities and assume the role of the physician. It explains how the doctor-patient relationship is established and outlines how the interview and the physical examination are performed. The method of organizing clinical data in the medical record is described. Finally, the book discusses how this information is analyzed in terms of the differential diagnosis of disease, the evaluation of the patient, and the planning of future studies and management.

THE ROLE OF THE PHYSICIAN

Role refers to the rights and obligations regulating the relationship between two people. The prescribed role of the physician entitles him to make personal inquiries of the patient, to examine his body, and to carry out treatment; but at the same time, the physician is obliged to be medically competent and to provide help and comfort. Correspondingly, a person in the role of patient is entitled to ask for a physician's help, to submit to examination without fear of exploitation, and to share in confidence his personal feelings and thoughts. Such a role confers upon him the obligation to cooperate with the physician and to accept the restrictions required for adequate study and treatment.

The codification of these roles provides the basis for the ethical and moral standards of medical practice. So basic are the principles regulating the relationship between physician and patient that many of the rules set forth in the Hippocratic Oath, though formulated almost 2500 years ago (460 B.C.), still have relevance for the physician today:

> I swear by Apollo Physician, by Asclepius, by Health, by Panacea and by all the gods and goddesses, making them my witnesses, that I will carry out, according to my ability and judgment, this oath and this indenture. To hold my teacher in this art equal to my own parents; to make him partner in my livelihood; when he is in need of money to share mine with him; to consider his family as my own brothers, and to teach them this art, if they want to learn it, without fee or indenture; to impart precept, oral instruction, and all other instruction to my own sons, the sons of my teacher, and to indentured pupils who have taken the physician's oath, but to nobody else. I will use treatment to help the sick according to my ability and judgment, but never with a view to injury and wrong-doing. Neither will I administer a poison to anybody when asked to do so, nor will I suggest such a course. Similarly I will not give to a woman a pessary to cause abortion. But I will keep pure and holy both my life and my art. I will not use the knife, not even, verily, on sufferers from stone, but I will give place to such as are craftsmen therein. Into whatsoever houses I enter, I will enter to help the sick, and I will abstain from all intentional wrong-doing and harm, especially from abusing the bodies of man or woman, bond or free. And whatsoever I shall see or hear in the course of my profession, as well as outside my profession in my intercourse with men, if it be what should not be published abroad, I will never divulge, holding such things to be holy secrets. Now if I carry out this oath, and break it not, may I gain for ever reputation among all men for my life and for my art; but if I transgress it and forswear myself, may the opposite befall me.[1]

Clearly, the oath recognizes the power of the physician inherent in the doctor-patient relationship and serves as a warning to him against its abuse. Fundamental to this relationship is the need of the patient to be able to place himself under the care of the physician with complete trust and confidence. Indeed, so potent is this need that patients commonly ascribe qualities and capabilities to their physicians which they do not, in fact, possess. Experience shows that the physician who is primarily motivated by concern for the welfare of his patient is not only less likely to abuse this trust, but he is also more likely to provide conditions conducive to an effective relationship. Francis Peabody aptly summarized this essential quality of a physician in his classical article, by saying, "the secret of the care of the patient is in caring for the patient."[2]

The desire to help others and to alleviate suffering which underlies the career choice of most medical students also helps them to assume the role of a physician as they begin their clinical work. When a student feels concern for the patient, he is already beginning to act like a physician. This is true even at a time when he has few skills and even less knowledge. It is common for patients to ascribe the role of a physician to the

---

[1]Jones, W. H. S.: Hippocrates. William Heinemann, London; G. P. Putnam's Sons, New York, 1923, Vol. 1, pp. 298-301. (In Greek with English translation.)

[2]Peabody, F. W.: The Care of the Patient. J.A.M.A., *88*:877, 1927.

student, simply because he wears the familiar white coat, carries a stethoscope, and is seen in the company of physicians. *However, most important of all is the student's expression of genuine, sustained interest in the problems and well-being of the patient.* This is what provides a realistic basis for the patient's feeling of confidence and his consequent willingness to cooperate. It is mainly through such interactions that the rights and obligations of the physician and patient are defined for the student.

THE DOCTOR-PATIENT RELATIONSHIP

The general consideration of the roles of the physician and patient does not define the nature of the relationship between any one physician and patient. This is determined more by the circumstances of the illness, the personal characteristics of the physician and of the patient, and the previous experiences of each. By no means are all of these determinants either conscious or rational on the part of either. The attitude of each toward the other may be based as much on personality characteristics, prejudices, or unconscious mental attitudes as upon the reality of the situation. Hence, consideration must be given to some of the factors that affect the first meeting of the student and patient and that influence the subsequent relationship.

Factors Influencing the Patient's Behavior

HIS NEED FOR HELP

When a person admits to himself that he is sick, he is conceding that he is no longer as self-sufficient as before. It is this acknowledged need for help which places him in the role of a patient and provides the opportunity to establish a doctor-patient relationship. People differ in their ability and willingness to accept the patient role. Some can accept dependency with ease and readily initiate a relationship with the student. But, if the dependent needs of such a person are abnormally great, he may also have unreal expectations of the student-physician, and may become anxious, angry, or depressed when such expectations are not fulfilled. Other people find the passive, dependent role threatening. For them it is very difficult to be a patient and to place themselves in the hands of a physician. They are prone to minimize or deny symptoms, to refuse to accept the usual hospital regulations, and may even display hostile behavior when the physician attempts to interview and examine them. Familiarity with the varieties of personality structure is of considerable aid in understanding how different patients relate to a physician.

HIS PAST EXPERIENCES IN THE PATIENT ROLE

Previous experiences with physicians, good and bad, will obviously influence how the patient relates to a new doctor. Yet, even when the patient's reactions are based primarily on the incompetent or tactless behavior of a former physician, it is notable how readily he will respond to the more adequate behavior of a new physician.

HIS PAST EXPERIENCES IN RELATING TO OTHER PERSONS

Very basic attitudes about accepting a physician's help originate from the patient's experiences with important persons in his childhood. The patient who as a child had confidence in his parent's capacity to provide help usually can place himself in the physician's hands with trust and confidence. On the other hand, a childhood experience with unreliable, rejecting, or neglectful parents may seriously interfere with the patient's capacity to have confidence in even the most dedicated physician. Such a patient may remain aloof, suspicious, and be only indifferently cooperative. Patients with an unfulfilled need for parental approval may try to gain the physician's acceptance, even by omitting or distorting facts.

It is, therefore, important for the physician to inquire about the patient's early and current relationships. By understanding how he interacts with others, the physician can anticipate the form that the patient's relationship will take, and he can modify his own behavior accordingly.

HIS FEARS CONCERNING THE ILLNESS

Some patients have major fears about the nature of the illness or of hospital procedures. Whether such concerns are realistic or not, the physician must recognize their existence and encourage the patient to speak of them. This often serves to overcome what might have been a serious barrier to communication. For instance, the patient who is afraid that his symptoms of cough and expectoration mean cancer will more readily talk if the physician discreetly inquires about his fears.

SOCIAL, CULTURAL, EDUCATIONAL, AND ECONOMIC DETERMINANTS

These factors may all significantly influence the patient's expectations of the physician. Especially when the student-physician's background differs from that of his patient, it behooves him to learn about the patient's upbringing and current life situation. The most immediate and practical means of so doing is through proper attention to the patient's personal and social history. (See Chapters 3 and 5.) Students who have had experience with people of backgrounds different from their own are at a decided advantage in this regard.

Factors Influencing the Student-Physician's Behavior

HIS INSECURITY IN THE NEW ROLE

A serious obstacle to the student's initial efforts to relate to his patient is his feeling of insecurity because of inexperience. Commonly, this leads to inappropriate diffidence on his part. The beginning student need not behave as if it is an imposition to inquire into the patient's illness or to perform a physical examination. He need not approach the patient apologetically to ask permission to carry out necessary tasks or to thank the patient for cooperating. *The student should appreciate that his personal educational goals and the patient's need for help are complementary, not antagonistic!* In fact, the opportunity for the patient to tell his story, to share his concerns, and to be examined by an understanding clinical student often is of therapeutic value to the patient. The student should also recognize that his ready access to other members of the clinical staff is an important means of communication for the patient. Further, the student is likely to spend more time with his patient and to know more about him than do many members of the staff. Blumgart illustrates the high degree of confidence a patient may develop in a student with the story of a patient who refused to consider surgery for severe gastric hemorrhage despite the advice of the Chief of Medicine and other specialists.[3] Only when the patient had a chance to talk it over with the fourth year clerk, did he consent to surgery! *The obvious lesson is that most patients regard the student as an important source of help. When the student acts accordingly, he will be more successful in establishing the type of relationship that will further his own learning and will provide the patient with the best type of care.*

HIS YOUTH AND INEXPERIENCE

This is not as much of a barrier in establishing a relationship as many students might think. There are some patients who, because they fear authority, may confide even more readily in a student than in an

---

[3]Blumgart, H. L.: Caring for the Patient. New Eng. J. Med., *270*:449, 1964.

older physician. A subtle factor that sometimes influences the patient's response to the youth of the student may be his relationship with his own children. For example, an occasional older patient may treat the student as a son whom he helps by providing the history and cooperating in the examination. A patient may even take pleasure in his young doctor's performance. An adolescent patient may perceive the student as an older sibling to whom he more readily can relate than to the older physician. On the other hand, it must also be appreciated that irrational attitudes on the part of a patient may derive from conflicts with his own children or with younger siblings, a fact which may become evident from how the patient speaks of his own children.

HIS PERSONAL ATTITUDES AND PSYCHOLOGICAL PROBLEMS

Each student will quickly discover that there are certain categories of patients with whom he readily gets along, and therefore likes, and others with whom he has difficulties, and dislikes. These attitudes involve such varied aspects of the patient as his age, sex, educational background, physical attractiveness, racial origin, and behavior. Predisposition to such biases on the part of the student is embedded in his own background and involves his personality, his unresolved psychological conflicts, and his prejudices. Such characteristics can be diminished through understanding and self-discipline, but usually can not be totally eliminated. When a student becomes aware of difficulty with a particular type of patient, it is well for him to try to understand what it is about the patient that disturbs him, so that he can attempt to modify his own reaction. For example, the student may find himself becoming irritated with a patient whose slowness and inattention hinder his obtaining a good history. Appreciation that such "stupidity" or "resistance" on the patient's part may actually reflect depression or organic brain disease, and is really not directed toward him as an individual, enables the student to overcome his feeling of irritation and to modify appropriately his approach to the patient.

While positive feelings toward a patient generally facilitate the establishment of a relationship, they should be questioned if they are exceptionally intense or if they are repetitively aroused by a certain type of patient. Under these circumstances, there is a risk of inappropriate involvement with the patient. Generally, such intense involvements have as their source some unresolved problem in the student. One is well advised to remember that no human being is free of the capability of behaving irrationally. Hence, when he finds himself intensely involved with a patient or when an instructor calls his attention to the inappropriateness of his reaction, the student should give some thought to what might be responsible and, if necessary, seek advice. Many times the problem is alleviated by discussing the situation with a more experienced physician.

THE CLINICAL SETTING

The student's first experience in the study and care of patients generally takes place on a hospital ward. Later he has opportunities to see patients in other settings, such as the out-patient department, the emergency ward, the community clinic, and even in the patient's home or the physician's office. The ward has many advantages for the introduction to clinical work. Patients are readily available, they are usually hospitalized long enough for unhurried study, and there is an ever-present professional staff for guidance and instruction. William Osler, the master clinician, may be credited with bringing the student from the lecture room to the patient's bedside in the teaching of clinical medicine.[4]

The Ward as a Clinical Laboratory

The student on the ward learns through actual experience and practice the role and functions of a physician as well as the nature, manifestations, and treatment of disease. He learns something of how illness and hospitalization affect patients and their families. He sees how doctors, nurses, nursing assistants, physical therapists, occupational therapists, social workers, technicians, and clergymen work with each other and with the patient toward the common goals of diagnosis and treatment. The student learns how to fit into this complex social structure. Above all, he learns how the physician makes observations and how he collects, records, and analyzes the information obtained from the patient, the family, and the laboratory. He also learns how such data are used to gain an understanding of the patient and his illness, which provides the basis for a plan of treatment.

The student discovers quickly enough that patients admitted to a hospital are likely to have serious or complicated illnesses. Even though he is a beginner, he no longer has the advantage of starting with the elementary and progressing to the complex. His first patients may be as difficult and as obscure as any he will encounter in the future, taxing the ingenuity and knowledge of his most experienced teachers. Often the

---

[4]Osler, W.: Aequanimitas with Other Addresses. The Blakiston Co., Philadelphia, 1952.

student will find serious disagreement among the staff as to the findings, their interpretation, and the management of the case. The thoughtful student appreciates the educational value of such disagreements. He attempts to learn the reasons for the conflicting opinions by inquiring of the staff and by studying the hospital record. He follows closely the subsequent course of events, attempting to form his own judgments. He observes his patients daily; he takes note of new findings; he follows his patient to the operating room or to the autopsy table; and when the occasion permits, he inquires about his patient's condition after discharge.

At the same time, the student will discover that often the hospital ward is a difficult place in which to work. There may be inadequate space around the bed. There may be poor lighting, interruptions by ward personnel, and noise from neighboring patients or low-flying airplanes. The patient may be away from the ward for tests. A student must learn to be flexible and adjust to such variable and frustrating conditions.

The Ward as a Social Structure

For both the patient and the student, introduction to a hospital ward requires adjustment to the rules, customs, and organization of an unfamiliar social structure. The new student adapts more quickly to the hospital setting if he is assigned to a specific area for a number of weeks. It is helpful for him to be conducted about the ward by a member of the staff and to be introduced to the personnel. He should also inform himself concerning the regulations and ward staffing routines, such as meal times, nursing shifts, and visiting hours. Some of this information may be posted on bulletin boards. Beyond that, the observant student, by tactfully observing the conduct of the various professional staff, quickly becomes familiar with the organization and his place in it. As this is accomplished, he finds himself in a position to observe what being in a hospital means to the patient.

Hospitalization is by no means a uniform experience for all patients. Some see it as a haven to which they come for help and the relief of symptoms; others see it as a strange and frightening place where they may be hurt or even die. But for all patients, admission to the hospital, especially for the first time, requires a major adjustment. They are separated from home and family; for some this may be distressing; for others, a relief. Patients are deprived of certain personal liberties and freedom of action, yet are relieved of many responsibilities. They are often confined to bed, and clothing and personal possessions are taken away. The schedule of meals and sleep is altered; there is a limited choice of diet. Unpleasant or painful procedures are anticipated, and distressing sights and sounds may be witnessed. At the same time, patients are provided with care and service; and are supported by the hope that their distress will be relieved and their problems solved.

In addition, patients find they must relate to a bewildering number of people. Even the active, well person in everyday life is not ordinarily called upon to meet, recognize, and relate to so many others and in such rapid succession. The nursing staff shifts three times a day; the house staff, medical students, and nursing students are rotated away from the ward; and consultants, dietitians, and technicians come and go. Anxiety, depression, irritability, anger, or other psychological disturbances may at times reflect the patient's inability to identify who is responsible for his care. It is in this area that the student may be particularly helpful. Because of the time he spends with the patient, often he is the most consistent person to whom the patient can relate.

The nurses, doctors, and students all share a responsibility for helping the patient adjust to the ward routine. *The basic principle involved is to reduce uncertainty as much as possible for the patient.* By being thoroughly familiar with the organization of the ward and knowing the names of the head nurse, the house staff, and the attending staff, the student can assist appreciably in orienting the patient to his new environment. *The student should also be sure to clearly identify himself and explain his own role in the future study and care of the patient.* As best he can, the student learns in advance what procedures, examinations, or consultations are planned, since, on occasion, he must inform the patient and explain the studies to him. Such preparation spares the patient the distress of the unexpected and often enables his questions to be answered or his fears to be resolved. The student also has the responsibility to inform his patient when he is to be presented on teaching rounds, to explain to him what is involved, and to answer any questions he may raise.

A subtle and often overlooked influence in a hospital ward is the effect patients may have on each other. Particularly in multibed units, the newly arrived patient may be indoctrinated by his roommates, not always appropriately. Patients come to know one another and often are distressed when their fellow patient gets sicker, is discharged, or dies. A patient's loneliness may be increased when his roommates have attentive visitors; or he may become upset when the others behave inappropriately. *The student must be attentive to the impact that other patients and their visitors have on his patient.* He should know the medical condition of others in the room, should observe how the patients interact, and pay attention to what each says about the other.

THE RESPONSIBILITIES AND OBLIGATIONS OF THE CLINICAL STUDENT

The primary objectives of the medical student are to learn the substance and methods of medicine and to achieve the professional role of the physician. These are best accomplished through graduated and carefully supervised engagement in the care of the sick, an activity which imposes additional responsibilities and obligations on the beginning student.

Obligations to the Patient

Under all circumstances, the well-being and comfort of the patient take precedence. He must be treated with respect and consideration in a professional, not in a diffident or apologetic manner. This means that the student has the right to interview, to examine patients, and to carry out certain procedures; and he should proceed to do so without apology. He must be aware that observations he makes do have relevance to the care of the sick, and that the great majority of patients expect him to carry out his duties in a business-like fashion. Most patients appreciate that the young doctor has to learn and are tolerant of the student's slowness or awkwardness. For the student, the factors which facilitate his work with the patient are sensitivity and concern for the patient's well-being. This, coupled with a professional attitude, does much to help the patient accept necessary but disagreeable procedures.

The professional attitude literally means that the student behave in a manner which patients expect of a physician. This includes attention to such matters as personal dress, grooming, cleanliness, language, and decorum, the standards for which are well established in the minds of patients. It means that gum chewing, smoking, horseplay, laughing, joking, sitting on the patient's bed, and other behavior quite permissible in other settings is unacceptable and, indeed, may seriously interfere with the patient's ability to establish a relationship and cooperate in the examination. The professional attitude calls for dignity, seriousness, conscientiousness, and the exhibition of a genuine intellectual effort to understand the patient's problems. It requires that personal interests and feelings not be permitted to interfere with the immediate task at hand, the relief of the suffering of another human being.

At all times, the student must be aware that the sick person is preoccupied with himself and may subjectively interpret or misinterpret whatever the student may say or do. The student must be thoughtful in his choice of language when speaking with the patient and must be alert to what the patient may overhear, whether at the bedside or in a totally unrelated corridor conversation. Confiding to the patient one's own personal problems or concerns is inappropriate.

Strict observance of the patient's right to privacy and confidentiality requires that information be shared only with other professionally qualified persons. At times, the patient needs to be reassured that his statements will be kept in confidence. Demonstration of sexual interest or expression of personal disapproval have no place in the behavior of the student-physician. *Basic to professional conduct is respect for the patient, regardless of how deviant his behavior may appear to be.* Such an attitude on the part of the physician is not only in the highest ethical tradition of medicine, but it is also essential if he is to effectively carry out his functions. One must be reminded that in times past, victims of epilepsy, venereal disease, and mental illness were regarded as objects of moral opprobrium and beyond the province of the physician. Even now, the role of the physician in the care of patients with such problems as alcoholism, drug addiction, and sexual deviancy is only beginning to be clarified.

Obligations to the Patient's Family and Visitors

Consideration for the family and friends of the patient is also important. They are often anxious in the hospital setting and may have made the visit at considerable personal inconvenience. Their presence can do much to help the patient adjust to the hospital as well as maintain a link with the outside world. When the student finds a visitor at the bedside, he should introduce himself, establish the identity of the visitor, and learn how long he has been with the patient. If it is only a short time and the student's business is not urgent, he should arrange with the patient and visitor to return later at a specific time. On his return, the student informs the visitor of the approximate duration of the examination, asks him to wait in the visitor's lounge, and notifies him when he has finished seeing the patient.

The student may also be asked questions by visitors. When these involve issues about the patient's illness they should, in general, be referred to the physician primarily responsible for the patient's care, either the house officer or the personal physician. It is his responsibility to keep the family informed concerning the patient's condition. Should an unforeseen complication arise, the physician-in-charge immediately notifies the family. On the other hand, it is quite appropriate for the student to respond to inquiries that do not directly concern the patient's condition, such as information about hospital routine.

Because visitors may be disturbing as well as helpful to his patient, the student should make a point to learn who visits and who does not. The effect of family and friends on the patient's feelings is noted. *The student should also make it a practice to interview important family members, not only for additional information concerning the patient, but also because it often is helpful for the relative to be able to speak of his concerns about the patient.* Further details on the technique of interviewing relatives are covered in Chapter 3.

Obligations to Ward Personnel

Others on the ward play a vital role in patient care. Consideration for them and their responsibilities is of utmost importance. For example, to delay a patient's dinner in order to finish a lengthy examination disrupts the work of the Dietary Department and results in the patient's receiving a cold meal. Interruption of the nurses' chart rounds or of drug administration at the bedside are only justified in urgent situations. When planning an interview or a physical examination, the student should check with the head nurse or the ward secretary to learn when the patient will be unavailable because of diagnostic or therapeutic procedures. Nonetheless, interruptions by nurses to administer medications, by technicians to perform tests, or by house staff to carry out procedures are unavoidable.

The student should understand that the information he obtains from his observation of the patient or family may be of great importance. If he has any reason to suspect that he has discovered something not known to the staff, it is his responsibility to bring it to the attention of the house officer or nurse-in-charge. A new symptom or sign, the inadequate functioning of drainage or intravenous tubing, an urgent question or complaint by the patient, all should be reported promptly. By serving as a channel of communication between the patient and other personnel, the student performs a service for the patient and enhances his relationship.

THE RIGHTS AND PRIVILEGES OF THE CLINICAL STUDENT

Along with responsibilities and obligations go rights and privileges. The student's role in patient care is well recognized. The legal responsibility for his supervision is assumed by the educational institution in the form of his preceptors, who are licensed physicians. The following are some of the rights and privileges of the clinical student:

1. *To interview.* This includes access to personal, family, and social data that are not ordinarily proper subjects of inquiry in a nonprofessional setting.

2. *To perform a physical examination.* The student has the right to perform a complete physical examination, including the rectal and pelvic examination.

3. *To carry out minor procedures.* When a student has attained competence through supervision, he may perform such procedures as venipunctures, throat cultures, or the passage of nasogastric tubes.

4. *To ask for help.* It is essential for the patient's well-being and the student's education that he feel free to seek help from interns, residents, nurses, and attending physicians.

5. *To examine his patient's charts and records.* These include records from other hospitals, for which authorization from a responsible faculty member is usually required.

6. *To speak with other personnel responsible for the care of the patient.* Should the student need additional information, he should speak with such staff as the house officer, the consultant, the social worker, the physiotherapist, the occupational therapist, or the dietitian. The patient's private physician is an important source of information, with whom the student should not hesitate to communicate in person or by a phone call.

7. *To observe special procedures or examinations.* When others carry out procedures on an assigned patient, including surgery, the student may be in attendance. Courtesy, however, requires that permission be obtained from the physician carrying out the procedure.

8. *To request access to laboratory material for personal examination.* This includes the privilege of examining such material as x-ray films, electrocardiograms, electroencephalograms, and pathological specimens. With this privilege goes the right to ask for assistance in interpretation. On the other hand, it is not the student's prerogative to *order* such procedures.

THE QUALITIES OF THE IDEAL PHYSICIAN

There is no agreement as to the qualities of the ideal physician or how such qualities are to be developed. Medicine is a broad and varied field. There is a place in it for persons of many different persuasions. Undergraduate medical education should produce an undifferentiated physician; that is, one who has grasped what is basic and essential to all medicine, yet who has had the opportunity to apply such principles in a variety of more specialized areas. Such a physician can then develop in whatever direction his personal inclination and talents indicate. Regardless of the ultimate career choice, the following are offered as the qualities that best exemplify the characteristics of the ideal physician:

He is first and foremost humane. The ideal clinician deals not simply with the abstraction, disease, but with a fellow being in distress. He relates to his patient with empathy, which implies the ability to understand and appreciate how the patient feels without being distressed himself. The physician appreciates that all that bears on his patient's life, comfort, and happiness is properly a subject for scientific inquiry and observation. To deal with the disease alone and forget the patient is to fail as an able physician.

He is constantly observant. From the time the doctor first meets the patient, or walks into the room, he is studying him and his surroundings to learn clues to his disease, his personality, and the sources of his distress.

He uses a systematic approach. He trains himself in the interview and physical examination, as well as in his thinking, to follow an orderly sequence and not to omit important findings. Yet, he is not inflexible; he is prepared to meet the new or unexpected and to adapt his approach.

He knows and understands basic principles. He has learned that comprehension of the basic reasoning behind medical concepts and techniques greatly enhances his capacity to apply knowledge and to devise approaches to new and unfamiliar situations.

He uses reason in all his actions. Each step in diagnosis and management is thoughtfully considered. He knows that the physician who approaches a problem automatically, or routinely, may fail to help the individual patient.

He is aware of the limitations of his own knowledge and of knowledge in general. He constantly strives to extend his knowledge and to learn for himself the boundaries of generally established knowledge. He is at all times ready to seek the counsel and help of the more experienced and is not afraid to say "I don't know." He learns to think logically and to commit himself to a diagnosis. However, he appreciates that any commitment he makes to diagnosis or treatment is subject to revision on the basis of new information, and he does not hesitate to change his views under such circumstances. The welfare of his patient takes precedence over his personal pride.

He respects the information that comes from the patient. While appreciating variation in patient reliability, he recognizes that the patient is likely to be the best source of information concerning his own condition, with close family members or friends as important supplementary sources. He knows that data derived from the interview and the physical examination provide the basis upon which further laboratory and other diagnostic procedures are selected, and that ordinarily such procedures are used to *confirm, not make,* diagnoses. He has learned that the indiscriminate use of laboratory procedures is not only uneconomical, but also may be misleading.

He is a perpetual student. He has developed the sequence of *see-think-read,* then think and see again. He interviews and examines a patient, then reads about the issues bearing on his observations. He returns to the patient to extend and clarify his findings which he uses to plan further diagnostic and therapeutic procedures. He never underestimates his own ability to make a new and original observation.

References

Blumgart, H. L.: Caring for the Patient. New Eng. J. Med., *270*:449, 1964.

Jones, W. H. S.: Hippocrates. William Heinemann, London; G. P. Putnam's Sons, New York, 1923, Vol. 1, pp. 298-301. (In Greek with English translation.)

Osler, W.: Aequanimitas with Other Addresses. The Blakiston Co., Philadelphia, 1952.

Peabody, F. W.: The Care of the Patient. J.A.M.A., *88*:877, 1927.

Chapter 2
THE DIAGNOSTIC PROCESS

Diagnosis has two major objectives. One is to characterize the nature of the pathologic processes in scientific, impersonal terms. The other is to evaluate the consequence of these processes in the individual patient. Feinstein has proposed that the first be referred to as the disease and the second as the illness.[1] The diagnostic process ultimately leads to the classification of disease and the evaluation of a patient's illness, both of which provide a rational basis for estimating his prognosis and planning for his care. For example, the term "diabetes mellitus" refers to the *disease* present in all patients so diagnosed. But the term gives relatively little information concerning an individual's experience with diabetes. In order to understand an individual's *illness*, one must learn about the severity, duration, stage, and course of diabetes in that patient; the influence of his particular biological or psychosocial disposition on the diabetes; and the impact of the disease on his way of life.

The diagnostic process is the mental operation through which the disease is identified and the illness evaluated. The procedures utilized by the physician are the interview, the physical examination, and various technical diagnostic procedures. The interview, whether directed to the patient or to an informed observer, yields information, such as the patient's subjective sensations (e.g., pain, nausea, or shortness of breath), his feelings (e.g., apprehension, despair, or irritability), changes in appearance (e.g., swellings, pallor, or skin lesions), and alterations in function (e.g., constipation, paralysis, or inability to work). The interview also provides information concerning the past health of the patient and his family, his development and relationships, and the setting in which the illness arose. In the physical examination, the physician evaluates the condition of the patient's body and his behavior. Diagnostic studies, such as blood and urine tests, endoscopy, electrocardiography, or roentgenography, are used to extend the range of the physician's observations.

The clinical manifestations of illness are classified as symptoms and signs. *Symptoms* are the subjective sensations and changes in body or mental function which the patient or the inquiring physician regards

---

[1]Feinstein, A. R.: Clinical Judgment, Williams and Wilkins Co., Baltimore, 1967, pp. 24-25.

as abnormal. Such information is obtained through the interview. *Signs* are the abnormal findings that are detected by the physician in the physical examination.

The diagnostic process involves a systematic analysis of symptoms, signs, and related clinical data. The physician must decide first which findings are abnormal by comparing them to accepted standards and to the individual's previous status. He then attempts to interpret the symptoms and signs in terms of underlying morphologic, biochemical, physiologic, microbiologic, or psychosocial factors to make the diagnosis of the disease. Finally, he evaluates the personal experience of the patient in relationship to the disease to gain an understanding of his illness.

The diagnostic process involves six separate but interrelated considerations:

1. The identification of the abnormal findings.
2. The localization of the abnormal findings in anatomic terms.
3. The interpretation of the abnormal findings in structural and functional terms.
4. The consideration of etiology.
5. The classification of the disease.
6. The evaluation of the patient's illness.

THE IDENTIFICATION OF THE ABNORMAL FINDINGS

The physician's first task is to identify which symptoms and signs are abnormal for the patient under study. From the patient's perspective, a symptom always signifies an abnormal state. In some instances, his interpretation is obviously correct, as when the complaint is shortness of breath, nausea, bloody diarrhea, or memory loss. In other instances, the symptoms are based on misinterpretation of physiologic variants, as when a patient anxiously expresses concern about a minor skin blemish. Persistence of such concern, in spite of reassurance, constitutes a symptom in its own right usually indicative of a psychologic disturbance. But not all patients report even obvious changes. For psychological reasons some minimize or even deny symptoms which are alarming to other patients. Such symptoms must be elicited by the physician. For example, a patient may deny that he is short of breath, but upon questioning may reluctantly acknowledge that he no longer takes his customary walks because he does not enjoy them. Further inquiry may reveal that it is because he gets "a little winded." Here, the doctor's experience enables him to identify a subjective abnormality not acknowledged by the patient, which must then be evaluated by objective examination. Some abnormalities are not experienced by patients as unpleasant or as a source of concern. An obese person, for instance, who has wished to slim down, may not report a loss of weight caused by developing diabetes; or the progressive symptoms of a cough due to bronchogenic carcinoma may be dismissed as a cigarette cough.

Changes in the patient's way of life may also reflect an abnormality. A patient may alter his pattern of eating because it makes him feel better; for example, he may find that frequent meals alleviate his hunger pangs, not recognizing these as ulcer symptoms. A patient may change his job because the work imposes too great a physical or psychological demand; or he may marry or separate in an effort to resolve a personal conflict. Thus, different life patterns may not only reflect a patient's response to some underlying physical or psychological disturbance, they may also constitute an attempt to alleviate or resolve the difficulty. The knowledge and the experience of the physician enable him to recognize when such changes in behavior are manifestations of disease.

Abnormal signs are observed by the physician during his examination. If obvious, the patient may also be aware of an abnormality that is asymptomatic, such as the growth of a mole or the swelling of his ankles. In general, the patient's symptoms alert the physician to look for abnormal signs. Once a physical finding is discovered, the physician must decide whether it is a physiologic variant or the product of disease; and whether it is related to the patient's present problem. For example, the enlarged thyroid of a patient raised in the iodine deficient goiter belt is of far less significance than an enlarged gland in a patient with symptoms of thyrotoxicosis; or the elevation of blood pressure on an initial physical examination has less meaning compared to the finding of sustained hypertension on repeated examinations.

Finally, other abnormalities are neither reported by the patient (symptoms) nor become apparent to the physician on observation (signs) but are discovered by means of laboratory tests or special diagnostic procedures. For example, red blood cells may be seen in the urine on microscopic study, a polyp in the sigmoid colon upon sigmoidoscopy, or an unsuspected lung lesion found in a roentgen film of the chest.

THE LOCALIZATION OF THE ABNORMAL FINDINGS IN ANATOMIC TERMS

Here the physician considers whether the abnormal symptoms and signs can be localized in terms of anatomic subdivisions of the body. It is convenient to think in terms of several different levels of organization:

1. A region of the body (e.g., the abdominal cavity or thorax).

2. An organ system (e.g., the gastrointestinal tract or a subdivision, as the terminal ileum).

3. An organ (e.g., the liver or heart).

4. Multiple systems (e.g., cellular structure or a tissue component, as the red blood cell, blood vessels, or connective tissue).

In general, one can readily assign symptoms and signs to the larger anatomic categories; namely, a region of the body, an organ system, or a specific organ. Symptoms or signs deriving from cellular or tissue abnormalities involving several organs or systems may be more difficult to recognize from the interview and physical examination alone. Special laboratory procedures may be required in such diseases as polyarteritis nodosa, hemolytic anemia, or multiple myeloma.

Once the physician decides on the gross anatomic location responsible for signs or symptoms, he progressively explores the finer morphologic divisions. For example, the patient may complain of chest pain. By appropriate questioning, the physician will attempt to localize the pain to a given organ or organ system. Does chest pain originate in the chest wall (related to body movement), the esophagus (aggravated by swallowing), or the heart (brought on by exertion)? If he determines that the pain is pleuritic by demonstrating its relationship to breathing, the physician will then try to determine the exact location by physical examination. For example, he will look for a pleural friction rub and underlying pulmonary findings. A chest film may help to pinpoint the diagnosis.

It must be appreciated that psychologic symptoms may also be expressed in bodily terms. The physician may suspect that the chest pain is psychologic in origin, such as a conversion symptom. He will then attempt to demonstrate that the pain does not fit any anatomic pattern and will investigate what psychologic factors are responsible for the choice of the chest as the location of the pain in that particular individual.[2] Whether the underlying basis is physical or psychologic, the location of a symptom or a sign does not necessarily correspond to its source of origin. Paralysis of an arm may not be a result of injury to the arm itself, but may be due to conversion or brain injury; vomiting may be caused by an emotional disturbance or by digitalis intoxication with no organic gastrointestinal basis.

Finally, it must be appreciated that some clinical manifestations, such as fever, generalized weakness, and weight loss, have no localizing significance. Such symptoms in themselves are of little help in making a specific diagnosis, but they do serve to indicate generalized or systemic involvement and may be a measure of the severity of the illness.

---

[2]Engel, G. L.: Conversion symptoms. *In* MacBryde, C. M.: Signs and Symptoms. Applied Pathologic Physiology and Clinical Interpretation. 5th Ed., J. B. Lippincott Co., Philadelphia, 1969, Chap. 26.

THE INTERPRETATION OF THE ABNORMAL FINDINGS IN STRUCTURAL AND FUNCTIONAL TERMS

The symptoms experienced by the patient and the signs observed by the physician derive ultimately from alterations in structure and function. Accordingly, the physician must analyze the relationships between signs and symptoms and interpret them in terms of underlying pathologic anatomy (e.g., inflammation, neoplasia, degeneration); pathophysiology (e.g., left ventricular failure, renal insufficiency, hepatic failure); or psychopathology (e.g., conversion, delirium, psychosis). This step in the diagnostic process carries the thinking of the physician from the primary clinical data to an explanatory level. The clinician must infer from symptoms and signs the abnormalities in function and structure. For example, from the findings of dyspnea, orthopnea, and rales at the lung bases he infers pulmonary edema.

Necessary for such diagnostic thinking is a thorough grasp of the preclinical disciplines and continued familiarity with advances in clinical science. It is most important to appreciate that the patient's account of his illness represents an attempt to put into words his awareness of changes in his body, in his mind, or in the external environment. As the physician listens to the patient's story, he attempts to visualize what is going on in terms of his own scientific knowledge. For example, a sudden pain increasing within 15 or 20 seconds to a peak intensity that is maintained for a minute or two, that then subsides, only to recur again in another minute, should evoke in the listener's mind the image of a peristaltic contraction meeting resistance. The ability to visualize mentally this physiologic process is dependent on the physician's knowledge of the innervation and motor behavior of smooth muscle in the walls of hollow viscera. From the location and radiation of the pain, he is also able to infer which hollow organ is the most likely site of the obstruction. Knowledge of the natural history of pathologic processes is then brought to bear on the clinical data in order to reach a conclusion concerning the underlying abnormality—whether, for instance, the obstruction is more likely due to a stone, a neoplasm, or a fibrous band.

Not only must the patient's symptoms be understood in structural and functional terms, but so must the abnormal physical findings. For example, the signs of neck vein distention, rales, and ankle edema, together with the symptoms of dyspnea and orthopnea, are interpreted to mean abnormal cardiac function or congestive heart failure. Physical examination can also pinpoint a structural abnormality, such as a heart murmur, that may not be known to the patient, and hence, not mentioned in his story. Finally, laboratory studies are introduced to confirm and quantitate abnormalities in functional and structural terms. Cardiac catheterization, for instance, will measure the degree of restriction of cardiac output, and angiocardiography will visualize valve thickening and immobility.

THE CONSIDERATION OF ETIOLOGY

In the final analysis, disease may be conceptualized as a failure of the organism to cope with forces originating within itself or its environment which disrupt its dynamic steady state.[3] The abnormal signs, symptoms, and laboratory findings may reflect damage as well as attempts to prevent or repair damage. The combination of forces which are ultimately responsible for such reactions of the organism may be considered to be the causes or the etiology of disease.

In considering the problem of causes, the distinction between the disease and the illness assumes particular importance. With respect to the abstraction, disease, it is often possible to make definitive statements about etiology. Indeed, the names of certain diseases are based on specific etiologic factors. For example, the disease, tuberculosis, is named after the tubercle bacillus, and the diagnosis is based on the isolation of the organism or the demonstration of the characteristic pathological changes. One is justified in saying that the cause of the disease, tuberculosis, is the tubercle bacillus. But such a statement would be inadequate in defining the etiology of the illness, tuberculosis, which is the experience of an individual infected with tubercle bacilli. The analysis of causes, therefore, must include not only the identification of specific pathogenic agents, but also an evaluation of the factors responsible for the patient's exposure and vulnerability to such agents. The latter may range from genetic or constitutional factors to social conditions. With respect to the causes of illness, medical knowledge is still very limited. It is easier, for example, to identify the tuberculosis organism and diagnose the disease, than to answer why the organism is localized to a given area of the body, such as the lungs, kidneys, or meninges, or to explain why the patient developed the disease at a specific time in his life. But it must also be appreciated that medicine not only is imperfect in its knowledge of factors accounting for the patient's illness, but that it also lacks knowledge to explain the specific etiology of many diseases as well, such as diabetes mellitus, hypertension, or peptic ulcer.

Since the physician deals with an individual patient, he must attempt to

---

[3]Engel, G. L.: Psychological Development in Health and Disease. W. B. Saunders Co., Philadelphia, 1962, Chap. 23 to 25.

elucidate the causes of the illness, not simply of the disease. In practical terms, this means that he evaluates all possible factors which might play a role in the illness. He inquires into genetic predispositions; early injury or developmental failures; exposure to microorganisms, toxic materials, or physical agents; and any underlying factors that may alter resistance, such as age, nutrition, alcoholism, or other disease processes. He learns of the condition of the patient's life and evaluates it for possible psychological stresses that may ensue from real or threatened losses, conflicts, or personal frustrations.[4] In a case of pulmonary tuberculosis, for example, a full statement of the causative factors might include a strong family history of tuberculosis with frequent exposure in childhood; and a current setting of depression, alcoholism, and malnutrition, precipitated by the patient's reaction to the death of his wife.

THE CLASSIFICATION OF THE DISEASE

Once consideration has been given to etiology, the physician attempts to classify the disease process. Because of imperfect knowledge, the nomenclature and taxonomy of diseases are quite arbitrary. The lack of knowledge is admitted in the names of some diseases, such as essential hyperlipemia or idiopathic thrombocytopenic purpura. Vague terminology may derive from historical tradition. Raynaud's disease, Hodgkin's disease, or Parkinson's disease are named after the men who first described the condition. On the other hand, Christmas disease (Factor IX deficiency) is named after the first patient in whom the disease was recognized. Initial colorful descriptive nomenclature has been retained in other diseases: lupus erythematosis (the condition of the red wolf), named after the reddish facial skin lesions; pernicious anemia (deadly anemia), because of the former uniformly fatal course; or gout (drop), because it was once believed that a noxious agent dripped into the joint to cause the disease.

In the past, characteristic symptoms and signs of diverse etiology were grouped together as clinical syndromes. With more precise diagnosis, the number of syndromes have declined. A few are still popular, such as Horner's syndrome, the nephrotic syndrome, or the chronic brain syndrome. Even the major divisions of systems of classification are heterogeneous and imprecise. Some diseases are listed according to the organ system (diseases of the cardiovascular system, liver, or kidneys); others are classified in functional terms (metabolic diseases, nutritional diseases, or demyelinating diseases); and still others according to eti-

---

[4]Engel, G. L.: Psychological Development in Health and Disease. W. B. Saunders Co., Philadelphia, 1962, Chap. 26 and 27.

ology (infectious diseases, diseases due to chemical agents, or hereditary disorders).

Obviously, such terminology is highly confusing. The student is best guided in the classification of disease by his textbook reading or special publications.[5] When making a diagnosis, he should try to be as precise and specific as possible. Syndromes or functional abnormalities, such as congestive heart failure, uremia, or anemia, must be defined further as to cause. When descriptive terms are used, they should be clear and complete; and if alternative nomenclature is available, the use of historical names should be avoided. Known specific etiologic agents are also included. For example, instead of saying Addison's disease, it is better to state "chronic adrenal insufficiency due to adrenal tuberculosis"; or "acute pneumococcal pneumonia of the right lower lobe" is more specific and preferable to "pneumonia."

THE EVALUATION OF THE PATIENT'S ILLNESS

The final step in the diagnostic process is to understand the effect of the disease on the individual patient. The severity of an illness makes it unique for that individual. In order to estimate severity, the abnormal findings are evaluated in quantitative terms and are compared to those of a person in a normal state of health. Symptoms, such as pain, dyspnea, or anxiety, are estimated with regard to intensity, rate of development, and duration. Physical findings are measured against accepted standards (e.g., the size of a mass is expressed in centimeters; or cyanosis is described as mild, moderate, or severe). The degree of structural or functional impairment is estimated in absolute terms (e.g., the range of motion at an arthritic joint), or in relation to the patient's previous capabilities (e.g., the amount of activity possible without fatigue or dyspnea). For certain diseases, standards have been established by committees of experts. For example, cardiac function ranges from Class I, with no symptoms, to Class IV, with symptoms at rest.[6] Important, too, are the character and magnitude of the etiologic factors (e.g., the virulence of the organism or the amount of radiation) and the condition of the patient at the time the disease develops (e.g., the degree of malnutrition or the presence of depression). One must not only evaluate findings in

---

[5]Thompson, E. T., and Hayden, A. C., Eds.: Standard Nomenclature of Diseases and Operations. Published for the American Medical Association by the Blakiston Division of the McGraw-Hill Book Co., New York, 1961.

[6]Criteria Committee of the New York Heart Association, Inc.: Nomenclature and Criteria for Diagnosis of Diseases of the Heart and Blood Vessels. P. F. Mallon, Inc., New York, 1955.

quantitative terms, but must also be aware of any discrepancies in the severity of symptoms and signs. For example, is the dyspnea out of proportion to the demonstrated findings in the cardiac and respiratory systems? Is the patient's professed inability to carry on his job as a carpenter in keeping with the demonstrated degree of anemia? Attention to such discrepancies is important, for it encourages the physician to consider alternative explanations.

Especially important, and often disregarded, are psychological and social factors. Knowledge of them is essential for a full understanding of an illness in order to insure proper management. Included are the patient's feelings about being ill, about being hospitalized, and about his physician; his concerns about finances, his family, or job; and the availability of family or friends for emotional support. Knowledge of the patient's personality structure is also important in order to determine what program of care will best meet his needs. For example, a diabetic whose life has been marked by planning, orderliness, and attention to detail can be expected to follow a rigid schedule of treatment by himself; he may be contrasted to the basically dependent, overdemanding, and helpless diabetic who will need continuing guidance and supervision from his physician. Or a cardiac patient, whose life pattern has been characterized by independent activity, may respond to an overly strict regimen of bed rest with so much restlessness and anxiety that he defeats this plan of care.

Information bearing on psychosocial factors is derived from the doctor's direct observations of the patient as well as from the reports of the patient and others that describe his manner of dealing with comparable circumstances in the past. For example, a patient's relationship to his physician may be predicted from knowing how he relates with others when he is in a dependent role. The patient who has had unrealistic expectations of his parents, his wife, or his boss is likely to expect magic from his physician; the patient who generally has been suspicious and lacking in trust in all of his relationships may be expected to display a similar attitude toward his physician.

*****

The diagnostic process is one of the greatest challenges in medicine. It tests the physician's power of logic and reasoning, and should be as scientific as isolating an enzyme in the laboratory. With the advance in medical knowledge and a better understanding of the etiologic factors in a patient's illness, the steps in the diagnostic process will become more explicit. Regardless of the future developments in medicine and therapeutics, the management of the patient extends far beyond the inoculation, the administration of a drug, or the transplantation of an organ. Essential to the patient's proper care is an understanding of the personal and environmental factors in his illness, which will always be a major responsibility of the physician.

References

Criteria Committee of the New York Heart Association, Inc.: Nomenclature and Criteria for Diagnosis of the Heart and Blood Vessels. P. F. Mallon, Inc., New York, 1955.

Engel, G. L.: Conversion Symptoms. *In* MacBryde, C. M.: Signs and Symptoms. Applied Pathologic Physiology and Clinical Interpretation. 5th Ed., J. B. Lippincott Co., Philadelphia, 1969, Chap. 26.

Engel, G. L.: Psychological Development in Health and Disease. W. B. Saunders Co., Philadelphia, 1962, Chap. 23 to 27.

Feinstein, A. R.: Clinical Judgment. Williams and Wilkins Co., Baltimore, 1967, pp. 24-25.

Thompson, E. T., and Hayden, A. C., Eds.: Standard Nomenclature of Diseases and Operations. Published for the American Medical Association by the Blakiston Division of the McGraw-Hill Book Co., New York, 1961.

Chapter 3

THE APPROACH TO THE MEDICAL INTERVIEW

The purpose of the medical interview is to obtain the historical information which the physician needs to make a diagnosis of disease and to understand the patient's illness.[1] Equally important, the interview serves to establish a relationship between the physician and patient. The information obtained by the interview is ultimately organized into the following five major categories:

1. *Present Illness* refers to the recent changes in health that led the patient to seek medical attention.
2. *Past Health* constitutes an overall appraisal of the patient's general health prior to the Present Illness. It includes descriptions of all illnesses and diagnosed diseases in the past.
3. *Family Health* covers the health of the entire family, living and dead, with particular attention to possible genetic and environmental determinants of disease.
4. *Personal and Social History* includes information on the development, life experiences, and personal relationships of the patient.
5. *The Systems Review* summarizes, in terms of body systems, miscellaneous symptoms that are not included in the Present Illness or Past Health.

The full content of these divisions and how they are derived from the interview data are discussed in Chapter 5. The physician uses the order of the written history only as a rough guide in conducting his interview. He keeps in mind the necessity to obtain information relevant to each of the five major categories but follows the patient's associations in the interview, exploring each manifestation as it is introduced, regardless of which category it will ultimately be assigned to in the write-up. Only after all the information has been obtained is it organized in the format of the medical record.

This chapter outlines the order in which an interview usually develops and describes the procedures to be followed to yield the most

[1]See Chapter 2 for the distinction between disease and illness.

complete information from the patient and other informants. The chapter also considers commonly encountered technical difficulties and how the interview need be modified according to the patient's illness.

The principles of interviewing are illustrated in Appendix A, including a verbatim transcribed interview and a running commentary on procedure.

THE CONDUCT OF THE INTERVIEW

No two interviews follow precisely the same course. Nevertheless, there is a common basic pattern, as follows:

Step 1: The physician greets the patient, introduces himself, and defines his professional role.

Step 2: He explores how the patient is feeling at that moment and takes any appropriate measures to make him as comfortable as possible before proceeding further.

Step 3: He invites the patient to mention all symptoms and complaints leading to the hospitalization (Present Illness).[2]

Step 4: He examines in detail the manifestations of the current illness, including the sequence of development of each of the symptoms, their characteristics, and their interrelationships (Present Illness). At the same time he listens for and follows-up the patient's spontaneous references to concurrent life circumstances, illnesses in the past, and issues of family health and relationships (Past Health, Family Health, Personal and Social History).

Step 5: He inquires in detail into the patient's past health, beginning with items already mentioned (Past Health).

Step 6: He inquires in detail about the family members, beginning with those already mentioned, and explores their health as well as their past and current relationships with the patient (Family Health, Personal and Social History).

Step 7: He explores the patient's current life situation and past development, beginning with items the patient has already mentioned (Personal and Social History).

Step 8: He systematically surveys symptoms on a regional basis (Systems Review).

Step 9: He inquires whether the patient has anything to add or questions to ask, checks the accuracy of certain important details, and informs the patient of the next step in the work-up.

The logic of this sequence derives from the psychology of the sick person who seeks medical assistance. (See Chapter 1.) For the patient,

---

[2]The term in parenthesis indicates the category in the written history under which information in this phase of the interview will be organized.

the goal is the alleviation of distress and the restoration of health. To accomplish this, he must first establish a relationship with the person who is to care for him. He must satisfy himself that this person is not only professionally competent, but is also interested in him as an individual. For the physician, the primary objective is to secure the information needed to understand the illness and to institute appropriate treatment. To achieve this, he too must initiate a relationship and gain the confidence of the patient. This he does by actively demonstrating his professional concern for the patient and by willingly listening to the patient's personal and medical problems. Until the patient feels sure of the physician, he may withhold or even distort important information lest it jeopardize the physician's opinion of him. For this reason, giving the patient the opportunity to express himself freely at the beginning of the interview assures fuller and more accurate information. These principles are evident in the sequence of the interview:

Steps 1 and *2* are designed to clarify the professional role of the physician and to communicate from the outset a genuine concern for the comfort and well-being of the patient.

The relatively unstructured inquiry of *Step 3* permits the patient to express himself in his own words, which gives the physician an opportunity to learn something of the patient's personality, as well as to hear what is of most concern to him. It also provides a general overview of the scope and variety of the patient's problems.

In *Step 4* the physician begins to make explicit the kinds of information he wishes, while still remaining responsive to the spontaneous associations of the patient. It is during this phase of the interview that both parties usually achieve an understanding of what each seeks from the other, and the detailed sequential history of the current illness is obtained.

The fuller exploration of Past Health, Family Health, and Personal and Social History *(Steps 5, 6,* and *7)* is pursued as the patient's confidence in the physician becomes established. The physician initiates his inquiry about more personal matters by referring to the patient's earlier spontaneous associations. In this way he respects the patient's right to speak of such issues in his own way and at his own time. The physician thereby avoids being intrusive yet demonstrates his interest in whatever the patient has volunteered about his personal or family life.

Finally, *Steps 8* and *9* bring the interview to a close and cover items which may have been either overlooked or misunderstood by the patient or physician.

Before discussing the actual procedure involved in each of these steps, a few words about note taking and tape recording are indicated. Each person will develop his own technique of note taking. As long as the patient feels he has the student's complete attention, taking notes does not interfere with the interview. It should be done as unobtrusively as possible. On occasion, it is helpful to explain to the patient why notes are being taken and to ask his permission.

Beginning students will find note taking an invaluable aid. By jotting down the salient points, the student will find it easier to keep the material straight in his mind. Especially when the history is complex, note taking makes it easier to listen to the patient's account without feeling overwhelmed, since the student can always quickly refer to his notes to remind himself of the material that has been covered. Notes need only be fragmentary, just enough to refresh one's memory when writing the history. Only occasionally are specific quotations called for. The seven dimensions provide the most practical guide for note taking (see p. 35). One records symptoms and events with the corresponding dates and times. Chronology is the most practical framework around which to organize notes. It enables the interviewer to see at a glance which periods of time have been covered and which remain to be explored. Key words or phrases may be used to designate the other dimensions. The names of important people and places are jotted down, along with ages or associated symptoms and events. If a sensitive area is being discussed, it is wise to discontinue note taking temporarily. A few minutes later, when the patient is on more neutral ground, notes can be made about the earlier material. Once a relationship with the patient has been established, the student should not hesitate to stop and scan his notes; this is less disturbing to the patient than to repeat questions already answered or to refer to inaccurate information. By and large, patients respect this as an effort to be complete and accurate.

In some of the teaching sessions, use may be made of the tape recorder. *The patient's consent must always be obtained before the interview begins.* He should be informed that the interview is to be tape recorded to make it possible to review the interview in detail later, perhaps with a senior doctor. He should also be assured of confidentiality. Only very exceptionally do patients object. Questions usually are concerned with who will have access to the tape. The microphone should be placed as close to the patient as possible, while the recorder itself is located so that the patient is not distracted by the moving reels. Should the student sense that the tape recording is interfering with the interview, its use should be discontinued and the patient so informed.

Step 1: Introducing One's Self to the Patient

Before meeting his patient the student first learns his name and proper title, whether Mr., Dr., Mrs. or Miss. He then introduces himself by name and explains that he is a student doctor helping the staff care for patients on the ward. He informs the patient that he is one of the group responsible for his care and wishes to speak with him about his illness. The beginning clinical student often finds it awkward to assume such a professional role. However, he can be assured that most patients readily accept him as a member of the professional staff and are more than willing to cooperate. Indeed, it is through this repeated experience of being accepted as a physician that the student's professional identity begins to evolve. It is neither necessary nor appropriate for a student to ask the patient's permission to be interviewed or examined.

After having introduced himself, the student should inquire whether it is a convenient time for the patient to be seen. It may be necessary to postpone the interview briefly if the patient has just been examined by the intern, is about to eat or go to the bathroom, or if he is awaiting medication for a distressing symptom. Aside from being common courtesy, such an inquiry is evidence of the student's concern for the patient's comfort and facilitates his acceptance of the student as a professionally responsible person. The introduction may be accompanied by a handshake. If the patient is too ill, the student may place his hand on the patient's arm or hand, which will initiate a physical contact and indicate personal concern. The patient's response to the introduction and to the handshake often imparts important clinical information as well (e.g., the cold, moist hand of the anxious person, the feeble grasp of the seriously ill person, the hearty handshake of the person who is denying illness, or the bewildered expression of the demented person).

Step 2: Putting the Patient at Ease

The first consideration is to be sure that both the patient and the interviewer are as comfortable as possible. The student assists the patient to get settled and then locates himself so that the patient can easily see and talk with him. Lights and window shades are adjusted so as not to shine in the patient's or student's eyes. In a multibed unit the curtains are drawn around the bed to give more privacy. It should be recognized that even with the curtains drawn, other patients in the room may be listening and the patient's confidences may be jeopardized. Therefore, when personal information is being discussed, it may be necessary to take him to another room or to postpone this part of the interview. If necessary, other patients in the unit are asked to turn down their radios or to speak more softly. Throughout the interview the student watches for the development of patient fatigue or other discomfort in order to intervene appropriately.

The patient is often preoccupied with his own immediate distress and will be gratified to know that the interviewer also shares this concern. Hence, the student's first questions should determine how the patient is feeling at that time: "How are you feeling?" or "How are you?" The inquiry is not intended to be a social amenity, and the patient is encouraged to respond accurately. He may answer by saying "Fine" or "Pretty good," which is rather inappropriate for someone who is sick. The interviewer's echoing, mildly disbelieving question "Fine?" or "Pretty good?" or "How do you mean that?" generally will lead to further elaboration by the patient. Whatever the patient's response, he should be encouraged to go into more detail. He may mention a symptom of his illness or may report that he has some unrelated discomfort, such as pain from an intravenous needle, or that he is cold, thirsty, or needs to void. He may refer to some aspect of being a patient, perhaps voicing concern about his family or his fear of the hospitalization. The student demonstrates his concern and interest by paying serious attention to what the patient reports. Whenever possible, he should make the patient more comfortable, perhaps by adjusting the intravenous tubing, by providing a blanket, or by offering the patient a glass of water.

The patient's response to the initial inquiry may indicate the degree of his physical discomfort and often tells something about his personality. His response is a guide to the further conduct of the interview. If he is in distress, he should be advised to keep the interviewer informed how he is feeling as the interview proceeds, so that it may be interrupted, shortened, or even postponed. When in doubt about the advisability of proceeding with a patient who is very uncomfortable, the inexperienced student should consult a house officer. An occasional patient, when asked how he is feeling, will generate a barrage of complaints about the hospitalization or express concern about his family or his job, which he had to leave without adequate planning. The patient should be given the opportunity to voice his concerns. Not only does this indicate the student's interest in the patient's problems, but also what is said is likely to include important information about the patient's personality and life situation. Failure to take the time to listen may be interpreted by the patient as a lack of interest on the part of the interviewer, and the result may be a perfunctory and uninformative interview. The student should also be alert to any discrepancy between the patient's answer and his appearance. Such discrepancies must be taken into account in evaluating the accuracy of the patient's story. For example, an obviously ill patient with a need to deny weakness or disability may answer "I'm fine." In his further reporting of the history, he may omit or distort symptoms and mislead the interviewer. Or, another patient may be smiling as he states he is suffering excruciating pain. This may be the response of an hysterical patient or of a patient who is exaggerating the pain to impress the doctor with his courage.

Step 3: Establishing the Major Areas of Complaint

This is a gross screening process which is best initiated by a general question, as "Will you tell me what led you to come to the hospital?" or "What has been the problem that brought you here?" The initial response to this type of question varies widely. It may be a defensive "What would you like to know, doctor?" "My doctor sent me" or "I don't know." It may be a single word or phrase, as, "pneumonia," "pain," "shortness of breath," or "nervousness." It may be a detailed account of an illness or simply a repetition of what the referring physician told him.

Whatever the response, the primary objective is to get the patient to indicate his immediate problem in broad outline. No attempt is made at this juncture to elicit the details. These will be fully investigated later. The student's first questions are designed to encourage the patient to speak freely. Whenever the patient hesitates or stops, he is invited to continue by echoing his last word or phrase in a questioning tone, e.g., "You felt nauseated? Uh-huh" or by saying "Yes?" or "And then?" or "Anything else?" The student is particularly attentive to the patient's report of symptoms and indicates his interest by a nod or by repeating the patient's phrase, as "Pain in your leg, yes. . ." When the patient finally appears to have completed his preliminary account, he is asked "Are there any other problems?" or "Do you have any other symptoms (or troubles)?" Such questions are repeated until the patient has nothing further to add. At some point early in the inquiry the patient's age should also be determined.

Obtaining this initial information may be compared to locating the major landmarks on a map or blocking out the rough outlines of a painting, the finer details of which are filled in later. Ordinarily this phase of the interview occupies 5 to 10 minutes and yields the following:

1. A list of all the symptoms and complaints which the patient considers to be important. Occasionally an articulate and well-organized patient will give an accurate and virtually complete account of his illness.

2. A demonstration of the patient's capability to express himself when given relatively little guidance by the interviewer. For example, he may be lucid, garrulous, inarticulate, or disorganized.

3. An indication of the patient's personality and how he relates to the interviewer. For example, he may be self-assured, independent, helpless, aggressive, shy, or evasive.

The initial list of symptoms and the patient's manner of reporting indicate to the student how he should proceed with the interview. At the same time, this nondirective approach assures the patient that he is free to discuss his problems. *To begin questioning about details before this phase of the interview has been completed may seriously interfere with the further conduct of the interview.* Until the student has an overall view of the patient's problems, he has little basis on which to judge how symptoms are related or which are the most important. This is particularly true when symptoms are due to more than one disease. For example, a patient may have two kinds of abdominal pain, one due to an active peptic ulcer and the other to liver congestion secondary to heart failure. The unwary student, inquiring prematurely about the details of the "pain," may not realize that the patient is confusing two types of pain. When later he discovers this, he has to go back and repeat the questioning in order to resolve the confusion.

An even more serious consequence of premature questioning is that the patient may be so distracted by the questioning that he forgets to report certain symptoms or assumes the student is not interested. For example, a patient coming for surgical repair of a hernia may have planned to say that he is also having a recurrence of peptic ulcer symptoms. If the student immediately focuses on the hernia problem, the patient may forget to describe his ulcer symptoms and go to the operating room with this fact unknown to the staff.

The manner with which the student approaches the interview will determine the way the patient responds. If the interviewer begins with numerous, detailed questions, patients may respond by waiting silently for the next question and provide little spontaneous elaboration of their own. This places the entire burden on the student who struggles to think what next to ask the patient. Such interviews commonly degenerate into unproductive question-and-answer sessions. Students who make this error sometimes describe these patients as being uncooperative or uninformative, when in fact it is the student's technique that has inhibited the patient's spontaneity. It is far more efficient to encourage the patient to speak freely at the very beginning of the interview, using the material he mentions as the basis for further questioning. In practice, it is easier to guide a talkative patient into productive channels than one who is reticent. The entire course of the interview may be determined by how successful the student is in encouraging a free flow of information in these first few minutes. At the same time, it is important to recognize that the very talkative patient who wanders, or who provides excessive and minute detail, will need to be guided back to the pertinent issues. Also, other patients with a poverty of associations will need considerable encouragement to elaborate upon their problems. Some overly talkative or silent patients may be psychotic or suffering from organic brain disease.

Step 4: Delineating the Present Illness

The opening phase of the interview will have established the basis for communication between physician and patient and will have indicated the general areas for diagnostic consideration. Complaints such as shortness of breath, vomiting of blood, fever, anxiety, or headache, bring to mind possibilities as to where the underlying abnormalities may be located; what the disturbances in function or structure may be; and even what some of the etiologic factors may be. The interviewer will note that the reported symptoms tend to group together, constituting episodes of illness. He now has the task of characterizing each of these episodes and analyzing the relationship of one to another. He first tries to identify which episode is responsible for the patient's current clinical problem (Present Illness). This calls for a detailed and *sequential* reconstruction of the patient's most recent symptoms with careful attention to their development and characteristics. In the course of pursuing the interview, it will ultimately become clear which episodes properly belong in the Present Illness, and which represent past illnesses. When dealing with a well-circumscribed disease in a previously healthy individual, this presents no problem. However, a great variety of clinical situations may be encountered which are more complex, making it difficult to define the Present Illness. For example, the presenting symptoms may reflect: (1) more than one disease, such as pneumonia in a diabetic or acute appendicitis in a patient with cancer; (2) an exacerbation of a recurring disease, such as a flare-up of rheumatoid arthritis or of peptic ulcer; (3) a complication in a pre-existing disease, such as the occurrence of a pathological fracture and spinal cord compression in multiple myeloma or an intestinal obstruction in chronic regional enteritis; (4) a complication of treatment, for example, Cushing's syndrome in a patient being treated with corticosteroids or a hypersensitivity reaction to penicillin; or (5) a psychological reaction, such as depression or conversion in a patient being treated for some organic disease.

Because of this complexity of illness, the exploration of the presenting symptoms will commonly extend into the patient's current life circumstances, his past health, and the health of important family members. Thus, although the main objective is to elucidate the Present Illness, this part of the interview may contribute importantly to many other aspects of the medical history. Indeed, the subsequent investigation of the Family Health and the Personal and Social History is facilitated when the interviewer is able to refer to items the patient has already mentioned. Also, the patient's spontaneous association of his symptoms to life events may contribute to a better understanding of the present illness. For example, a patient's reference to his father's recent heart attack, while describing his own shortness of breath, may alert the listener to the possibility of a psychic origin of the symptom, namely conversion; or a patient with fever and abdominal pain, who comments that he has recently been in Mexico, raises the possibility of an amebic liver abscess.

Before discussing in more detail the interview techniques that are useful in delineating the present illness, it is necessary to describe how symptoms are characterized for diagnostic purposes and how the physician directs the interview yet simultaneously follows the patient's associations.

THE CHARACTERIZATION OF SYMPTOMS FOR DIAGNOSTIC PURPOSES

Symptoms, as elicited by the interviewer, are the patient's verbal expression of perceived changes in his body or mind. The physician's task is to reconstruct from the patient's words the bodily or mental processes underlying the symptom. To accomplish this, symptoms are considered in seven dimensions, as follows:

1. *Bodily location.* Where is the symptom located?
2. *Quality.* What is it like?
3. *Quantity.* How intense is it?
4. *Chronology.* When did the symptom begin and what course has it followed?
5. *Setting.* Under what circumstances does it take place?
6. *Aggravating and alleviating factors.* What makes it worse or better?
7. *Associated manifestations.* What other symptoms or phenomena are associated with it?

These seven dimensions are central to the diagnostic process. They provide the information which enables the physician to decide whether a complaint reflects an abnormality; and if so, where this abnormality is located and the nature of the underlying functional and structural disturbance. The student will find it to his advantage to commit these seven headings to memory, for they constitute the basis for the questions he will need to ask about each symptom.

Bodily Location. Most symptoms are localized by the patient to some region of the body. Where and how the patient localizes a symptom must be described accurately. Thus, the localization of a pain may be very precise or vague; it may spread or it may radiate; it may cover a large or small area; it may be superficial or deep.

Quality. Patients usually communicate quality by analogy. A symptom is described as being "like" something else. Either the patient selects a familiar experience, (e.g., "like whirling on a merry-go-round" to designate vertigo); or one which is based on his imagination, (e.g., "like being squeezed in a vise" to describe the chest pain of myocardial infarction). Some descriptions reflect underlying physiological or psychologic processes. For example, the expiratory wheeze of asthma clearly reflects the difficulty of expelling air through narrowed bronchioles. Other descriptions have been established by clinical experience and have no clear physiologic explanation, such as the crushing or squeezing chest pain of acute myocardial ischemia.

Quantity. The quantitative aspect of symptoms refers to (1) the intensity of the symptom itself (e.g., mild, moderate, severe, unbearable); (2) the degree of impairment of function, often estimated by changes in the person's everyday activities; (3) the frequency, (e.g., of urination, cough, bowel movements); (4) the volume, (e.g., of vomitus, sputum, hemorrhage); (5) the number, (e.g., of convulsions, ecchymoses, attacks of pain); (6) the size or extent, (e.g., of a rash, ankle edema, abdominal swelling).

Chronology. A precise reconstruction of the sequence of development of symptoms and events provides the best opportunity to understand the development of the underlying pathological processes. There are four major components to chronology:

1. ***The time of onset of symptoms.*** The exact time of the first symptom and of each subsequent symptom must be established as precisely as possible. The intervals between symptoms and their order of development also have important diagnostic significance. For example, mild malaise, followed over the next three months by weakness, weight loss, night sweats, and cough, culminating in hemoptysis, suggests lung cancer or pulmonary tuberculosis; in contrast, a day of malaise and slight cough, followed in the next 24 hours by a shaking chill, high fever, pain in the chest, and blood-flecked sputum, is more in keeping with an acute bacterial pneumonia.

2. ***The duration of symptoms.*** The duration of individual symptoms conveys important information about the underlying pathological processes. It must be established exactly whether a symptom extends over minutes, hours, days, weeks, or months. The duration of unconsciousness in syncope due to cardiac arrest, for example, is a matter of seconds or minutes at the most, since asystole longer than a few minutes would be incompatible with life. On the other hand, the weakness and fatigue of such disorders as pernicious anemia or hypothyroidism may develop slowly over months or even years.

3. ***Periodicity and frequency of symptoms.*** Symptoms usually are not constant, and their pattern of variation often reflects the rhythms or periodicity of the underlying pathologic processes. Thus, obstruction of a hollow viscus is associated with the rhythmic increase and decrease of pain (colic); the chills and fever of malaria are correlated with the life cycle of the parasite. Not only may the pathologic processes cause periodic symptoms, but they also may be affected in turn by periodic

phenomena, such as times of eating, sleeping, exercise, menstruation, work, or the regular weekend visits of in-laws. The pain of peptic ulcer, for instance, characteristically occurs during periods when gastric acid is unbuffered by food.

4. ***The course of the symptoms.*** The time course of a symptom also reflects the nature of the underlying process and must be explored with care. Does the symptom stay the same? Does it get better or grow worse over time? Does it remain the same for a long time and then progress rapidly? Or does it run a remitting or relapsing course? For example, a pain which builds up, reaches a peak, and then slowly subsides over the course of a minute or two, thereafter recurring every three or four minutes, is characteristic of the peristaltic contractions of a hollow viscus attempting to overcome an obstruction; a steadily increasing difficulty in swallowing is indicative of a developing organic obstruction of the esophagus, such as cancer, while intermittent difficulty in swallowing which does not progress suggests spasm.

Setting. At the time an illness or a symptom is experienced, the patient is always (1) somewhere (e.g., he may be at home, in bed, in his car, on the job, or on vacation); (2) doing something (e.g., he may be sleeping, eating, bending over, shoveling snow, or watching TV); or (3) in relation to some person (e.g., he may be with, or wish to be with, someone; or he may wish to get away from someone, such as his wife, his mother, his boss, or a police officer). In the very recent past he may have suffered a serious personal loss or a job frustration. He may have been exposed to a toxic substance or an infectious agent. Exploration of these factors helps the physician to understand symptoms as well as to characterize the patient. He learns how symptoms are embedded in the matrix of the patient's life; that is, how life activities influence the symptom, and how the symptom influences the patient's life.

Aggravating or Alleviating Factors. Understanding how a symptom may be influenced by certain activities or physiological processes helps to clarify the nature of the underlying problem. For example, straining, physical exertion, eating, or coughing may respectively aggravate the pain of peritonitis, coronary insufficiency, esophageal neoplasm, or pleurisy. On the other hand, lying still, resting, avoiding food, or breathing quietly are activities that may relieve the pain of each condition. The student can best think of aggravating factors as imposing a burden beyond the functional capacity of the affected organ system, while alleviating factors reduce the demand.

Associated Manifestations. It is rare to have only one symptom associated with a disease process. Not only will the malfunction of a given organ express itself in several ways, but also there are often systemic symptoms of general bodily dysfunction. For example, a patient with an infectious disease, such as pneumonia, often has the systemic symptoms of fever, sweating, and anorexia, as well as the localizing symptoms of cough and chest pain. With experience, one becomes familiar with *symptom complexes*, which are associations and combinations of symptoms characteristic for specific disease processes. Thus, it is important to know whether vomiting occurs without nausea, or nausea without vomiting, or whether the two occur together; or whether loss of weight is associated with increased appetite, with decreased appetite, with vomiting, with diarrhea, with pain, with feelings of depression, or with no other symptoms at all. Knowledge of anatomic and physiologic principles provides a guide to the association of symptoms. For example, loss of weight in spite of increased food consumption suggests the inefficient carbohydrate utilization of diabetes or the hypermetabolism of hyperthyroidism; whereas, gain in weight despite decreased food intake suggests the possibility of fluid retention.

All seven dimensions also have relevance to the characterization of symptoms caused by psychological and behavioral disturbances. Even bodily location is pertinent, as when a psychological symptom is expressed in physical terms, such as a conversion symptom, a hypochondriacal symptom, or a somatic delusion. In contrast to organically based symptoms, the other dimensions are more likely to be elaborated in psychological, interpersonal, or social terms rather than in physiological terms.

THE IMPORTANCE OF FOLLOWING THE PATIENT'S ASSOCIATIONS WHILE DIRECTING THE INTERVIEW

The necessity to delineate the illness and to characterize symptoms in the seven dimensions requires that the student provide direction in the interview. Encouraging the patient to speak freely continues to be the basic requirement for a productive interview, since only the patient can describe what he has been experiencing. On the other hand, he usually does not appreciate all that the interviewer needs to learn from him. In order to accomplish his task of diagnosis, the student must subtly direct the course of the interview. Far from being merely a passive listener, he indicates to the patient by his responses and questions the need for certain organization and content. The patient soon comes to appreciate that events must be dated, sequences established, and symptoms described precisely. At the same time, such direction must not be achieved at the expense of prejudicing the patient's responses or of blocking the free flow of his associations. The amount of direction needed in the interview varies with the patient. Some will wander and discuss unproductive areas in minute detail; others will gloss over important historical points, and still other patients will present a coherent story where little intervention is needed. It is most important that the student be flexible in his interview technique, learn to adapt to the patient's style of reporting, and still remain in control of the situation. The student should neither passively listen to volumes of irrelevant detail, nor should he conduct the interview in the manner of a courtroom lawyer by firing repeated questions. Obviously, much practice and experience are needed to achieve the proper balance.

The two objectives, to encourage the patient's spontaneous associations and to provide direction, are best achieved by always initiating the inquiry into each new area with open-ended (nondirective) questions and by following with progressively more specific (directive) questions until the subject is fully clarified. This means that the interviewer must have clearly in his mind what details are necessary to understand the illness yet not prematurely impose his ideas on the patient. For example, he may begin the investigation of a symptom with the request, "Tell me more about it" or "What was it like?" This allows the patient to say whatever he wishes about the symptom and to bring up his own associations, unprejudiced by the interviewer. The student, as he listens to the patient's account, is alert to omissions and ambiguities, and periodically indicates what needs to be clarified; e.g., "That was when?" "What was the feeling?" "Which came first?" As the patient completes his more spontaneous account, the interviewer then follows with whatever specific questions are necessary to complete the picture. *In so doing, he always tries to formulate each successive question on the basis of what the patient has just said.* In essence, just as is done in sustaining a conversation, the student picks up where the patient leaves off. By following the patient's lead, he avoids the disruption of the patient's train of thought and important associations emerge naturally under such conditions. When a series of direct questions are posed early in the interview, the patient may respond simply by waiting passively for the next question. Only when the interviewer is satisfied that he has obtained all the information that he needs by following the patient's associations, does he again take the initiative to change the subject and introduce a new topic. Each new area is pursued in the same manner. Thus, the interview typically consists of a series of interconnected sequences, each one of which begins with open-ended questions and progresses to increasingly more specific questions until the issues are fully defined.

Throughout the interview, the student remains attentive to the patient's spontaneous associations, even when at first they may seem to be irrelevant. The patient is allowed to digress long enough to establish whether the information is pertinent to the history. If so, he is encouraged to continue. *All the while, however, the student must keep in mind what information the patient has not yet clarified, so that he can return later to ask the necessary questions at an appropriate time.*

The value of pursuing the patient's associations is illustrated in the following example.

> A 34-year-old man, complaining of headaches, mentioned that they seemed to get worse toward the end of a day's work. When asked at that point what his work was, the patient described a job in a poorly-ventilated auto repair shop. Spontaneously, he began to wonder whether exhaust fumes could be responsible for the headaches. This was a plausible suggestion, since headaches are a symptom of carbon monoxide poisoning. Inquiry about working conditions, however, revealed this cause to be improbable. Asked what he did after leaving work, he said that he often procrastinated about going home, stopping at a bar to visit with his cronies. He went on to explain that he and his wife were not getting along well, so that often he was reluctant to go home. As he mentioned this, he began to wonder whether tension could have anything to do with the headaches. Further questioning about his marital situation, however, left no doubt that the headaches preceded the difficulty with his wife by several months. Asked about other circumstances when headaches occurred, he mentioned playing golf, working in his basement workshop, and romping with the children. Exploration now revealed that repeated bending over was the common denominator for all the situations in which the headache developed. This discovery suggested that a mechanical factor was important; and indeed, it turned out that the headache was due to a brain tumor.

In this example, each of the associations had to be examined in its own right. Some proved to be blind alleys in respect to the final diagnosis of brain tumor, but all yielded information important for a better understanding of the patient.

THE TECHNIQUES USED IN OBTAINING THE PRESENT ILLNESS

Initiating the Detailed Exploration of the Illness. The detailed inquiry about the current illness begins after the patient has given a general but brief account of his difficulties (*Step 3*). The student now must decide which aspect of the illness should be inquired into first. In general, one begins with the problems which are most recent and most urgent:

1. If the illness appears to be a circumscribed incident of recent origin, the student may start with such questions as, "Exactly when did this all begin?" or "What was the very first thing you noticed?"

2. When the patient has reported several episodes of illness or a series of attacks, it is usually best to begin with the most recent one. This is freshest in the patient's mind and usually most germane to his seeking medical attention. After the details of the most recent episode have been clarified, one explores the preceding episodes and the intervals between them. In this manner, all the earlier incidents are considered until the entire complex has been reviewed.

3. Sometimes the symptoms presented in the initial phase of the interview fall into no obvious pattern. Under such circumstances, the

best approach is to begin with whatever the patient has emphasized as most important. If it is unclear what this is, he may be asked "What has been the main difficulty?" The same approach is used when the patient indicates the existence of several problems simultaneously. For example, a patient might report several weeks of malaise, poor appetite, weight loss, diarrhea, and abdominal pain. He also may mention that his "sugar diabetes" has been out of control and that he has been "down in the dumps." Beginning with what appears to be the most urgent matter, all symptoms will have to be considered in turn and their interrelationship explored.

Using the Seven Dimensions as a Framework to Clarify the Illness. The seven dimensions, *Bodily location, Quality, Quantity, Chronology, Setting, Aggravating or alleviating factors,* and *Associated manifestations,* provide a frame of reference around which the interviewer proceeds to organize his inquiry. Because of many years of practice, the experienced physician is able to pursue these dimensions with little conscious effort as he listens to the patient's report of symptoms and is aware of any omissions or ambiguities. On the other hand, the beginning student must actively concentrate to keep all the dimensions in mind and to be sure that each symptom is fully clarified in terms of the seven dimensions.

The dimension which contributes most to the organization and clarity of the history is *Chronology.* Dates and times serve to anchor the history in such a way that relationships between symptoms and events can be more clearly seen. Hence it is good practice to inquire as early and frequently as necessary "When was that?" "When did that occur?" "What year (month, day, time) was that?" "Then what happened?" or "And then?" Such reminders serve to impress upon the patient the importance of times and sequences, encouraging him to pay more attention to chronology in his spontaneous account.

The techniques of exploring each dimension are discussed in the following paragraphs. There is no fixed order of exploration, and the student must keep in mind that he is trying to reconstruct the picture of the entire illness rather than merely a succession of isolated symptoms.

Bodily location. Generally, patients refer to bodily location in rather broad terms, such as "arm," "head," "stomach," or "back." The appropriate first question is "Where in your ____________?" or "What part of your ____________?" Many patients proceed to demonstrate the location; those who do not should be asked to do so. With such symptoms as weakness, dizziness, or gas, the patient may be asked "Where do you feel the ____________?" Whatever the patient's response to these first questions, the matter should be pursued further by first asking more open-ended questions as "Do you feel it anywhere else?"

"Does it go (radiate) anywhere?" and finally, if the information is not yet forthcoming, more explicit questions as "Did it involve this part of your hand?" (pointing) or "Did you feel it on the surface or deep?" or "Did it go through to the back?"

Quality. Inquiry as to the quality of the symptoms is usually best initiated by asking "What was (is) it like?" The patient is then encouraged to elaborate further. If he has difficulty or uses vague terms, like "hurts," "sick," or "dizzy," the interviewer helps him by asking, "What do you mean by ____________?" or "Was it like anything you have ever felt before?" If these questions are unproductive, he offers him a choice of terms: "By 'hurting' do you mean a pain, an ache, or what?" "Do you mean sick to your stomach, sick all over, or what?" If the symptom is a pain, he might ask, "Well, was it sharp, or sticking, or dull, or aching, or what?" without emphasizing one more than another. This encourages the patient to provide a suitable term of his own, or he may respond with strong agreement to one of the terms offered him.

Quantity. Questions concerning frequency, volume, number, or size may be approached quite directly, as "How many times did you vomit that night?" or "How much blood did you spit up?" Vague answers, as "A lot" or "Not much," are not adequate, and the patient must be encouraged to be more exact. "What do you mean by 'A lot'?" If the patient still is vague, he may be asked, "Was it two or three times or six or eight times?" "Did you bring up a few streaks of blood, a teaspoonful, or more than that?"

The intensity of a symptom and the degree of impairment of function are best estimated in more personal terms. "How bad (severe, serious) was it?" will encourage the patient to elaborate. He may then be asked to compare it to a previous experience: "Have you ever been this anxious before?" or "How does it compare to the worst pain you ever had?" Asking the patient to compare a pain to a toothache, to an injury, or to childbirth is a good way to estimate severity.

Functional impairment is best evaluated in terms of the extent to which the patient's pattern of living has changed as the result of the symptom or the illness. With a specific symptom, like dyspnea, dizziness, or stiffness of a limb, he may be asked what he is not able to do now that he could do before. Specific questions follow, such as "How many flights of stairs can you climb?" (dyspnea) or, "Can you button your jacket?" (paresis of the hand). With poorly localized symptoms, such as fatigue or anxiety, or when evaluating the overall impact of the illness, a useful approach is to have the patient describe in detail his activities on a recent day. A specific day, such as the day before hospitalization, is chosen rather than just a "typical" day. The latter often yields only a stylized report, lacking the small details that are so informative. For example, the patient may be asked, "Tell me what your day was like on Monday, from the time you got up until you went to bed." He may then be asked, "If you were well, what would your day have been like?" Obviously, such accounts also yield useful information about the patient and his current life situation, data which can be expanded further at that time or later on in the interview.

Chronology. *Every effort must be made to establish chronology in terms of calendar dates and clock times.* This requires a deliberate effort on the part of the interviewer, since people tend to keep track of time through events and circumstances that are important to them, rather than by calendar dates. Only through such associations do they establish the day or hour. Thus, a man will be sure that his pain began around 3 P.M. because it was shortly after his 2:30 P.M. coffee break; or he will recall that his first attack was at least 14 years ago because it was before his oldest son was born. The interviewer should use the same approach. Each time he asks "What date or time was this?" he should note the patient's reference points. He then uses the same points to guide him in clarifying time relationships. For example, "You began to feel sick to your stomach around 4 o'clock, while you were doing the laundry; did you vomit before you finished, or afterwards?"

On occasion, patients will spontaneously provide exact dates or times. It is always well to inquire how they remember the time so exactly, for not uncommonly it proves to be associated with some important event. For example, a patient may say without hesitation that his first episode of chest pain occurred at 7:15 P.M., March 3, 1967. He remembers the date exactly because that was the day he received word that his son was injured in an auto accident, and he remembers the time because the pain began while he was watching the evening news on TV.

Usually, patients have difficulty in accurately recalling dates. In the great majority of cases, the interviewer can resolve the uncertainty by reference to important landmarks. For example, the patient who can date the onset of illness no more accurately than, "a few months ago," may be asked how he was feeling during the Christmas holidays, during his summer vacation, or on his birthday. Familiarity with details of the patient's life is particularly helpful, for then one can refer to important specific events. For example, how was he before he moved, before he started his new job, after the baby was born, or while his father was in the hospital? Indeed, it is far easier for both the patient and the interviewer to establish the date of onset of symptoms and to keep accurate track of their sequence if they are related to concurrent events in the patient's life. Contradictions and discrepancies are more readily detected and corrected when the interviewer is able to make such comments as, "Earlier you said the pain began in January, but now you say everything was fine until a week after the baby was born. Wasn't she born on February 10th?"

By careful attention to such details, one will find that it is mainly the delirious, demented, psychotic, or mentally defective patient who is totally incapable of providing reasonably consistent dates and time relationships; indeed, their failure to do so with such an inquiry should suggest one of these diagnoses.

The date of onset of the illness must be accurately established and its entire course accounted for, right up to the time of the examination. This means that the student must investigate with great care the time of onset of the illness, and no subsequent time interval should be left unaccounted for during the course of the illness. Regardless of the point in time selected by the patient as marking the beginning of his first symptom, the student should always inquire how the patient was before that time. He must be explicit; if the patient reports the first symptom as beginning at noon, the student must inquire about that morning and the night before; if the patient dates the onset to January, he should be asked how he was during the Christmas holidays or on New Year's Day. Such questions are pursued until the patient clearly identifies a point or period in time when he definitely was feeling well. Some patients, by discounting earlier difficulties, are inclined to date the onset of the illness to the time when they first became concerned about symptoms. This tendency can be checked by inquiring whether the patient had in any way been previously restricted in his activities, or by asking, "Have there been times when you felt better?" He may then acknowledge that he had not really felt well for several months.

Having identified the time of onset, the interviewer then encourages the patient to give a sequential account of the illness and of each symptom. The frequent inquiries, "When was that?" and "Then what?" serve to reinforce for the patient the importance of accuracy of times and sequences. As the student listens to the patient's account, he makes mental note of time gaps, all of which must be accounted for in the history. With a long and complex illness, he will find it useful to jot down the sequence of dates covered so that he can check omissions before bringing the interview to a close.

At times it is important to establish as precisely as possible the duration of a symptom, for example, unconsciousness, where a difference between seconds and minutes may be crucial for the diagnosis. This is best done by having the patient reconstruct the surrounding events and estimating the probable time involved. For example, the patient may remember feeling dizzy, calling out to his wife, and then blacking out. He may next recall his wife coming toward him or someone carrying him into an ambulance. By establishing how long it would take for his wife to get to him, or for the ambulance to come, a fairly reasonable estimate of the duration of unconsciousness is possible.

Setting It is easy to clarify the setting if the student uses events in the patient's life as guides to evaluate functional impairment and to time the sequence of symptoms. Some patients will spontaneously interrelate their symptoms and concurrent events. Others, assuming that the doctor is not interested in personal issues, will give an impersonal account of symptoms. Patients can easily be induced to provide information about the setting if the student interposes such questions as "Where were you when this happened?" "Who was there?" "Who helped?" "What were you doing at the time?" The patient is then asked to elaborate. For example, a patient who reports an acute onset of shortness of breath and weight gain may at first answer the question "Where were you?" with "Home, asleep." In response to further questioning, he may reveal that he has been upset since his wife left him a month earlier; and because he has had to eat his meals at a nearby restaurant, he has not been able to follow his salt-free diet. From such a response, important information is obtained which bears not only on the illness itself, but also on the personal and social background of the patient. Later in the interview, these can be the starting points for further investigation of the Family Health as well as the Personal and Social History.

Finally, as diagnostic possibilities occur to the student, questions bearing on etiologic factors should be asked. For example, had the man with recurring chills and fever been in a malaria-infested region; had the farmer with acute respiratory distress been cleaning out a silo; or had anyone else at work been jaundiced? Direct questioning, on the other hand, is rarely informative in acute psychological disorders, such as an anxiety reaction or a paranoid panic. In these instances, the relevant precipitating circumstance is much more likely to emerge in the course of the patient's spontaneous account of events immediately preceding the episode.

Aggravating or alleviating factors. The first clues to aggravating or alleviating factors generally come from the patient's own account of what was going on when the symptom became better or worse. This again emphasizes the value of encouraging the patient to describe the circumstances as well as the symptoms of an illness. He may tell of awakening intensely short of breath and feeling better after sitting up; he may describe how the pain in his back suddenly increased when he tried to pick up his grandchild; or that his chest pain lessened after he stopped walking. Each such association is then examined further. The patient may be asked, "Is there anything else you found that helped, (made it worse)?" "What did you do to try to help it?"

Knowledge of clinical syndromes leads to more specific questions. Thus, the physician knows that the pain of angina pectoris develops while walking and subsides within a few minutes with rest, or that the vertigo and nausea of labyrinthitis are brought on by slight movements of the head. Questions should be worded so as not to influence the answer. Thus, when inquiring about angina, one asks, "What effect does walking have?" "Standing still or sitting down?"; or when asking about vertigo, "What happens if you move your head?" "How much movement will bring on the symptoms?"

Associated manifestations. The relationships between symptoms logically emerge in the course of developing their chronology. Nonetheless, it is still necessary to inquire directly into the nature of such associations, especially when the patient describes symptoms occurring in the past. For example, he may tell of dyspnea, orthopnea, and ankle swelling occurring "3 or 4 months ago"; and later speak of anorexia, nausea, and abdominal distress "2 or 3 months ago." In order to establish whether the gastrointestinal symptoms are related to those of heart failure (e.g., congestion of the liver and gut), a complication of treatment (e.g., digitalis toxicity), or an independent illness (e.g., conversion or gastroenteritis), it will be necessary to reconstruct the exact sequence of events.

Knowledge of clinical syndromes enables one to anticipate symptoms that the patient does not mention. If diabetes is suspected, for example, the student should inquire about polyuria and polydipsia; or if a pain is thought to represent conversion, he should ask about other symptoms of conversion, such as globus, hyperventilation, or episodes of paralysis and anesthesia.

The technique of characterizing symptoms may be summarized as follows: *The student keeps the seven dimensions in mind as the patient is allowed to tell his story in his own words. Incomplete information about any of the seven dimensions is noted, and the patient's attention is directed to these gaps, starting with nondirective questions, and following with specific questions, as necessary, until all the information is obtained. Throughout the interview, the student encourages the patient's associations, pursuing those which seem informative.*

The Wording of Questions. The basic principles determining the wording of questions are as follows: (1) the patient should have no difficulty understanding what is being asked; (2) the form of the question, while indicating what type of information is of interest to the interviewer, should in no way prejudice the patient's responses; and (3) the question should be so worded as to induce the patient to speak freely. To meet these requirements the following are essential:

1. Questions should be brief and simple. Whenever the student finds himself having to explain a question, he should stop and think through exactly what it is he wants to find out. The examples in the preceding text and in Appendix A illustrate the proper construction of questions.

2. The student should use language that is understandable to the patient. This will require taking into account the patient's level of edu-

cation and his background. It is particularly important to avoid the use of medical terms that may be unknown to the patient, such as pleurisy, jaundice, or paralysis. Instead, a brief description of the symptoms may be offered: "Did it hurt when you took a breath" "Did your skin ever turn yellow" or "Did your hand ever become so weak you couldn't use it?"

3. Only one question should be asked at a time. To string several questions together or to ask about more than one item leaves the patient uncertain as to what he should answer.

4. In exploring any issue, the inquiry should always start with nondirective questions, reserving more direct questions to fill in gaps, clarify ambiguities, or verify facts. Questions which can be answered with a simple "yes" or "no" should be used sparingly; otherwise, the patient may assume that little more is expected of him and fall into a pattern of silently waiting for the next question.

5. One should use the patient's own terms, at least until there is mutual agreement as to what the term means. Failure to do so may lead to confusion for both the patient and the interviewer. For example, a patient may refer to a sensation in the chest as a "pressure." The proper question is "Tell me more about the pressure sensation." For the interviewer to substitute some other word, such as "pain," may be a distortion of the patient's intent. It is especially confusing when the patient has reserved the word, "pain," for some other sensation.

Clarifying the Patient's Responses. It is often necessary to intervene and clarify what the patient is describing. Such expressions as "nervousness," "sick to the stomach," or "a funny feeling," usually have a quite personal meaning, and the student must inquire promptly what the patient means. Thus, it is misleading to the point of diagnostic confusion to assume that the patient's term, "sick to the stomach," means nausea, when clarification would have revealed that he really is referring to a sensation of fullness. Once the term has been clarified, it avoids confusion for the interviewer to actually use the patient's term in his further questioning: "Tell me more about being 'sick to the stomach'."

Medical or quasi-medical terms, such as "pneumonia," "tumor," "sciatica," or "nervous breakdown," must always be clarified, both with respect to the patient's understanding of the term and with respect to the details of the illness so designated. One is never justified in assuming that a name diagnosis, even if ascribed to another physician, is necessarily correct. The patient must always be asked to describe the symptoms and course of the illness in his own words. When a patient says he had an "appendectomy," for instance, the operation may indeed have been performed; but further inquiry may reveal that the history was more compatible with a conversion symptom or with regional enteritis than with appendicitis.

Some patients, when asked to tell about their illness, may omit symptoms altogether and persist instead in reporting what their doctor said and did. A patient with anemia, for instance, may give a detailed description of the medications that his doctor had given him or explain that the x-rays showed he had something wrong with his stomach, and so on. The interviewer should lose no time in making it clear that he is more interested in learning about the patient's symptoms. "Yes, I would like to know what Dr. Smith said, but first I want to hear in your own words how you have been." Occasionally, it is necessary to repeat this several times to remind the patient.

Should the thread of the story be lost, whether because the student was momentarily inattentive or because the account was disorganized, the patient must be interrupted. The interviewer should not hesitate to say "I didn't follow that" or "I'm not clear about this" and ask the patient to repeat or clarify his account. When he is consistently unable to present a coherent story, a diagnosis of delirium, dementia, psychosis, or mental deficiency is suggested.

Obtaining Essential Factual Data. Certain types of information must always be obtained and recorded as precisely as possible. The patient's account may have to be interrupted to complete such data. These include (1) the age and birth date of the patient; (2) the dates relevant to the illness; (3) the full name and location of previous physicians; (4) the dates of previous hospitalizations and the names of hospitals; (5) the name (or description) of medications, including the dosage and by whom prescribed; (6) the details of medical treatment; (7) the current ages of relevant family members or other important persons; (8) the dates of significant life events, such as births, marriages, divorce, job changes, or military service.

Pursuing the Course of the Interview. Although it is virtually impossible to predict how any interview will proceed, the student must appreciate that the process is by no means haphazard. Usually he tries to complete the investigation of a symptom or an event at the time the patient mentions it. He allows the patient to continue his spontaneous account as long as he seems to be bringing up information relevant to that symptom, and then he asks such questions as are necessary to fully characterize the symptom in its seven dimensions. Should the patient, in the context of describing the present illness, refer to a more remote illness or event, this should be followed up at the time, at least briefly. A patient may say, for instance, that he experienced similar symptoms several years ago when he had infectious mononucleosis. Then, he recalls that his father, who died of cancer of the stomach, had similar symptoms during his terminal illness. Not uncommonly, students will fail to obtain the necessary details of important information at the time the patient speaks of it. It may only take a minute or two to learn the essential facts of the patient's infectious mononucleosis or the father's age, date of death, and prior state of health before the terminal illness. The practice of briefly completing information as the patient mentions it not only takes advantage of the patient's willingness at the moment to go into more detail, but also indicates the student's interest in the material. Judgment must be used as to when one should round out the finer points of historical data so as not to interrupt the patient's train of thought. Failure to do so will necessitate the student's having to return and question the patient again in order to obtain a complete history. This not only lengthens the interview, but also may aggravate the patient who feels he has told all of this before.

After the essential information has been obtained, one returns to complete the material that has been interrupted. Sometimes patients will bring up two, three, or more items of importance in rapid succession. Here one has no choice but to select one topic first, but not without indicating interest in the other topics and informing the patient that he will want to know about them later. In all cases, the guiding principle is to invite the patient to tell the story in his own words and then progressively to direct him in such a way that the history is revealed with the least distortion.

Completing the Main Body of the Interview. This phase of the interview comes to a close when the interviewer feels that he has learned as much as he can about the present illness. With some complaints, such as an injury, a hernia, or an attack of renal colic, only a few minutes will be required. Most illnesses, however, will usually take the student 30 to 60 minutes to learn the necessary details. An experienced physician will need half the time. At this juncture, the following information usually has been obtained: a reasonably complete account of the presenting complaints and the events leading up to admission; namely, the Present Illness; some information about concurrent illnesses and illnesses in the past; and some information about the patient's personal history, including the important persons in his life.

Usually, at this point the interviewer is aware of a certain lull. The patient no longer is reporting spontaneously, and the student has run out of questions with respect to the current problems. Before he moves to the remaining sections of the history and performs a systems review, he must be sure that he has the following information which is appropriate to most present illnesses:

Pertinent positive and negative information. In considering various disease entities that might explain the patient's illness, the student should inquire about expected symptoms the patient may not have mentioned. For example, if lupus erythematosis is a consideration, the student may need to ask whether or not the patient has had a facial rash, convulsions, or pleurisy. The influence of environmental factors is also included in such questioning. If pertinent to the present illness, the possibility of infectious or chemical exposure must be considered. Has the patient traveled recently? Is there a similar illness in the family or at work?

Medications and treatment. What treatment has the patient received for his present illness? This includes physical restrictions, physiotherapy, prescribed exercises, and all medications that he is taking for this or for concomitant illnesses. The name and dosage of each drug, if not known to the patient, may be learned later from the referring physician or pharmacist. In particular, it should be remembered that patients may be taking analgesics, tranquilizers, sleeping pills, or oral contraceptives on a long-term basis. Finally, it is important to know who prescribed the particular treatment or medication, including whether it was the patient himself.

Weight. The patient should always be asked what his present weight is and whether there has been any recent gain or loss. The maximum and minimum weight in the past should also be determined.

Degree of disability. If not already known, the student should learn what limitations the patient's illness has imposed on him and his family. Such information is particularly important in chronic illnesses.

After the student has obtained what he considers a reasonably complete description of the illness, he shifts his attention to filling in the missing information relevant to the other parts of the patient's history.

Step 5: Investigating the Past Health

The inquiry into past health may be introduced by asking "How has your health been in the past?" Here, one is interested to learn about periods of good health as well as about episodes of illness. Since health is a relative experience, it is always necessary to clarify the patient's response to this question. Even "good" or "excellent" may hide significant symptoms or disability in the person who needs to see himself as strong and in control. Answers such as "pretty good" or "fairly good" should always be taken to indicate that there have been health problems. If the patient does not spontaneously elaborate, he should be asked "What does 'excellent' (or 'pretty good') mean for you?" One should inquire not only about the symptom, but also about what the patient's range of activity was like when well. "What were you able to do (or what was your life like) before you got sick?" is an effective way to evoke such a description.

An occasional patient counters the general question about his health with "Do you mean physical health?" This is his way of revealing the existence of emotional problems and is best answered with "I mean any kind of health problem."

Whatever the patient brings up as the result of this inquiry is then explored in more detail. It is important to have an adequate description to be able to accurately identify the illness, even though fewer details are needed than for the present illness. The student should learn the date of onset, the symptoms, the course, the treatment, and any sequelae. Names of physicians, the nature of diagnostic studies or of surgery, and the dates and location of hospital admissions are also noted. The student should investigate each past illness to be able to reach his own conclusion regarding diagnosis. The patient is asked to describe the illness in his own words; then specific questions may be needed to check the reliability of the diagnosis. For example, the patient who reports "gallbladder trouble" should be asked specifically about those manifestations of gallbladder disease that he failed to mention, such as jaundice, dark urine, or fatty food intolerance. *No diagnosis claimed by the patient, even when attributed to a reliable physician or medical center, should ever be accepted at face value.* There is always the possibility that the patient has misinterpreted information, or that even the most definite diagnosis may prove incomplete or wrong in the light of new information.

Sometimes the exploration of past health reveals that the present illness actually began earlier than the patient had previously indicated. For example, a patient may have described the symptoms of an acute myocardial infarction coming on in a period of "excellent" health. Later in the review of past health, he may mention a "muscle strain" that occurred six months earlier, consisting of aching pain in his anterior chest and left arm, and mild dyspnea during exertion, relieved promptly by rest. Without consulting a physician, he cut down on his physical exertion and the symptoms disappeared. He did not spontaneously associate these earlier symptoms with his present illness even though they were identical in location and character. Actually, these symptoms, angina pectoris, were the first manifestations of coronary heart disease and appeared six months earlier than the initial account of the present illness had suggested.

After the patient has been given an opportunity to tell about all the illnesses he can remember, the student completes the information in the following categories:

1. General health
2. Childhood health
3. Adult health
   a. Medical illnesses
   b. Surgical procedures
   c. Psychiatric illnesses
   d. Obstetrical history
4. Accidents and injuries
5. Allergies and immunizations

The inquiry is first a general one, beginning with questions such as "What childhood illnesses did you have?" "Have you had any other illnesses?" "Any emotional problems?" "Have you had any (other) operations?" "Injuries?" "Any problems during pregnancy or childbirth?" "Any allergies?" "Are you sensitive to any medicines or drugs?" More specific questions about each category of illness will need to be directed to the patient. For example, when he is asked "What childhood illnesses did you have?" one is not satisfied with the answer "The usual ones" but must inquire about important childhood illnesses by name. The question may need to be amplified to refresh the patient's memory. For instance, the student may need to clarify "rheumatic fever" by saying "Did you ever miss school for weeks or months because of illness?" "Did you ever have a prolonged fever that kept you in bed for several weeks?" "Did you ever have swelling or aching of your joints, frequent nose bleeds, growing pains, or St. Vitus' dance?"

Finally, one inquires specifically about illnesses which may have a bearing on the patient's current problem. For instance, inquiry about previous nephritis, urinary tract infection, or renal trauma would be important in a patient with hypertension or renal failure. In a patient with femoral artery insufficiency and intermittent claudication, one should ask about diabetes, previous foot infections, and other complications of atherosclerosis, such as coronary heart disease.

Step 6: Investigating the Family Health and Family Relationships

The student now shifts his attention to the family, asking about the health of each member and his role, past and present, in the life of the patient. In a well conducted interview, many of the family members will already have been mentioned, and a good deal learned about them and their relationship to the patient. One initiates inquiry into the family health by referring to one of these family members: "You mentioned that your wife is 43 and is working in a factory. How has she been?" If she has not been well, one should determine the nature of the illness, the degree of disability, and how the patient has been affected by his wife's illness. When asking about relationships, it is helpful to elicit the patient's feelings: "How did your wife's illness affect you?" or "How has the marriage been?" One then may inquire as to the length of the marriage and the wife's childbearing experience. This logically brings one to the children, each of whom should be identified by name, age, sex, state of health (present and past), present whereabouts, occupation, marital status, and children. When the patient's children are widely separated in age, one should always keep in mind the possibility that a parent may have remarried. In this manner, one progresses through the family, accounting for husband or wife, children, grandchildren, parents, grandparents, and siblings. One should also inquire whether any siblings or children have died, whom the patient may have forgotten to mention. Common-law partners or foster parents should be included. It is also pertinent to inquire about uncles and aunts where hereditary diseases are being considered. One should identify which family members are most important to the patient, since they are the ones whose health and activities will have the most bearing on the patient's status. At some point it is always well to inquire "Who is at home?" or "With whom do you live?" for this may reveal other persons of importance to the patient, such as in-laws, distant relatives, a common-law husband or wife, foster children, or friends. One may also learn from such a question that the patient is separated from his spouse or even living with someone else, a fact that the patient may have hesitated to volunteer.

Whenever changes in relationships with important persons are encountered, such as separations, illnesses, deaths, or retirement, dates should always be ascertained and the impact on the patient of such changes established. "How did this affect you?" or, if it is obviously distressing, "That must have been a difficult experience for you" usually suffices to bring out the feelings of the patient. In terms of understanding him and the possible implications for his illness, *how the patient reacted to the event is of far more importance than the event itself. It is not adequate merely to note the event without learning something of its effect on the patient.*

With respect to illnesses and deaths of family members, one should learn the diagnosis, the manifestations of each illness, and the age and date of death. There are at least two reasons why it is important to know the details of the family member's illness: First, it provides a check on the validity of the diagnosis reported by the patient. As an example, adequate questioning about the grandfather's "asthma" may make it evident that it was more likely congestive heart failure. Second, the manifestations of a family member's illness may have direct bearing on the patient's own symptoms. For example, if cough were a major symptom of carcinoma of the lung in the father, the fact that the patient's cough began on the anniversary of the father's death might suggest that it was a conversion symptom. Similarly, a patient with bronchitis, who knew his father died of carcinoma of the lung, may anxiously exaggerate how much he has been coughing or he may avoid mentioning it altogether, lest he discover that he too has carcinoma of the lung.

In bringing to a close the inquiry about family health, the student specifically questions the patient about diseases that might be related to his own illness through contagion, as in tuberculosis, or through a genetic factor, as in diabetes or epilepsy. It is well to remember that some inherited diseases may not be directly manifest in parents or grandparents. Hemophilia, for instance, which is attributed to a sex-linked recessive gene, may be clinically evident only in an uncle or male cousin. A good final question with which to conclude is "Has anyone in your family ever had an illness like yours?"

Step 7: Completing the Personal and Social History

By this point in the interview the student should have learned a good deal about the setting of the illness, the current life situation, and the family. If he has not, it is likely that he has conducted the interview in such a way as to neglect relating the illness to the patient's life. To introduce for the first time an inquiry into the personal and social background at this point in the interview is not likely to be productive, for it will be artificial and out of context. On the other hand, if the student has been following the course of the patient's illness in the context of his pattern of life and his family relationships, there will now remain only the task of filling in areas left unfinished earlier in the interview. Commonly, the patient's trust in the student has by this time matured to the point that he is quite willing, sometimes eager, to discuss personal concerns which he may have been hesitant to reveal earlier in the interview. These concerns may be of considerable importance for subsequent judgments about management and prognosis.

How fully each aspect of the personal and social history must be covered depends on the individual case. *In all instances, full information about the patient's current life situation is mandatory.* Beyond that, the patient himself generally indicates what is pertinent if the interviewer shows interest and follows the patient's leads. His age and the nature of the present problem give some indication as to what should be more fully explored. For example, information about early childhood is much more relevant in an adolescent or a young adult than in an elderly person. When emotional problems are prominent, a fuller exploration of the early life history is indicated, regardless of the patient's age.

The personal and social history aims to provide an overall perspective of the patient's adjustment and functioning over the years. The best way to assay this is to sample how the patient has dealt with developmental and other crises of life. Accordingly, one inquires into his performance and reactions under such circumstances as leaving school and home, military service, marriage, illness or death of important persons, or changes in his economic or social status. As already stressed, *emphasis is always on the patient's reactions and method of coping with these events, not simply on the event itself.* The interviewer's preconception of how stressful or significant an event is does not necessarily correspond with how it is perceived by the patient. Retirement, for example, may be a blessing to one person and an intolerable burden to another. Good general questions to ask whenever the patient reports some such change in his life are "How did this affect you?" or "How did you feel?" Dates and sequences are important to clarify the temporal relationship to past and present illnesses.

The details of important points in the Personal and Social History may be found in Chapter 5. The major subdivisions of the Personal and Social History are organized as follows:

CURRENT LIFE SITUATION

This covers information about *present* living arrangements and relationships to family and friends. Included are descriptions of the home and family, present occupation and economic status, social and community commitments, leisure activities, and the patient's personal characteristics and pattern of living. One emphasizes whatever may be current sources of concern to the patient and whatever may be important for his future care. Information from family or friends is also helpful in evaluating the current life situation.

PAST DEVELOPMENT

This category considers the patient's *past* personal and social history and is organized into three major subdivisions: childhood and adolescence, educational and occupational history, and marital and family history.

With respect to the interview itself, these personal issues are not dealt with in a categorical fashion. The attentive interviewer will learn a good deal just from what the patient chooses to discuss. For purposes of elaboration, the best technique is to begin with a general question referring to a major area of life experience. For example, "Tell me about your childhood" and "When did you first leave home?" are good questions to begin a discussion of childhood or adolescence. While much of the information concerning persons important to the patient, such as parents, children, husband or wife, will have already been obtained, additional details concerning relationships may emerge as the patient discusses his development. When one wishes to encourage the patient's responses, the best technique usually is to pursue information that is already known. For example, "You say you work in a bank. What do you do?" "Who is your boss?" "What was your job before that?" and so on, keeping in mind that one always follows the patient's lead and not a prepared set of questions. It is relatively easy to move from such a beginning and progress to related areas, such as schooling, military service, or outside activities, until a general outline of the patient's development and way of life has been obtained.

Obviously, new information about the present illness, past health, or family health may appear in this phase of the interview and should be pursued in detail.

Step 8: Reviewing Symptoms by Systems

The Systems Review serves to organize symptoms and signs in terms of the major systems of the body. It has two purposes:

First, it is used by the interviewer as a guide in elaborating symptoms of the patient's present illness. A complaint of chest pain, for example, should immediately suggest the need for a full review of the items covered under the Cardiovascular and Respiratory Systems. It is usually appropriate to do this at the time the presenting complaints are being investigated.

Second, the Review of Systems is used to inquire about symptoms and signs in the patient's past history that may have been overlooked in the interview. Specifically checking each system may uncover further symptoms of an illness already discussed or of an illness not yet mentioned. One may also encounter miscellaneous symptoms which do not fit into any particular diagnostic category or those which represent minor responses to psychological stress.

It is relatively easy to commit to memory the order and content of the Systems Review if one keeps in mind the several general headings and what symptoms result from specific organ dysfunction. The review proceeds systematically: Beginning with the skin and hematopoietic system one proceeds to the head and neck and down the trunk to the extremities, covering each of the major systems. Below are listed the general categories of the Systems Review. The specific items are found in Chapter 5.

Skin
Hematopoietic system
Head and face
Ears
Eyes
Nose and sinuses
Mouth, pharynx, and larynx
Breasts
Respiratory tract
Cardiovascular system
Gastrointestinal system
Urinary tract
Genital tract (male)
Genital tract (female)
Skeletal system
Nervous system
Endocrine system
Psychological status

Except when elaborating a symptom of the present illness, it is important that the direct questioning of the Systems Review be reserved for the very end of the interview. An inexperienced student may be tempted to shift to the Systems Review early when there is silence on the part of the patient or when the student feels he is running out of questions. Premature introduction of such a direct question-answer approach can serve to block the unfolding of the history by the patient, with consequent loss of important data. Whenever the student is at an impasse how to proceed, he may ask himself if he has thoroughly covered the course of the illness and evaluated the symptoms in terms of the seven major dimensions.

It is manifestly impossible to establish the occurrence of each and every symptom experienced by the patient in the course of his life. Although the Systems Review contains a great number of items, in practice, the interviewer asks a general question under each major heading and follows this with a rapid and brief query about those items that seem most relevant for the particular patient. In this fashion, he proceeds in an orderly manner through the whole sequence. Each positive response should be developed fully and its relationship to previously noted illnesses should be clarified.

An example of questioning in the Systems Review with respect to the respiratory tract would be "Have you ever had any trouble with your lungs?" "Breathing?" "Asthma?" "Wheezing?" "Cough?" "Do you cough up anything when you wake in the mornings?" "Have you ever coughed up blood?" "Ever have pleurisy, or a pain on breathing?" "Night sweats?" "When was your last chest film?" If the patient does not know what pleurisy means, an explanation must be given or a more colloquial term used. It is helpful, as the student progresses through the review of systems, to mention the names of common illnesses that the patient may have forgotten to mention; for instance, "Have you ever had pneumonia?" under the respiratory tract; "ulcer?" or "gallbladder trouble?" under the gastrointestinal system.

When a patient responds affirmatively, it is necessary to clarify whether the symptom reported represents an occasional and inconsequential manifestation (e.g., everyone coughs at some time), a normal physiological phenomenon (e.g., becoming winded after running), or whether it constitutes a significant change for him (e.g., dyspnea on climbing one flight). If the latter, the symptom should be evaluated briefly in terms of the seven dimensions.

Occasional patients respond positively to virtually every question. This is an important finding, especially in a patient who earlier described his general health as "pretty good." It may indicate a psychological illness (conversion or hypochondriasis), or be a clue to multisystem disease not heretofore recognized. Other patients minimize complaints and need to be pressed to bring out the information. Thus, a 55-year-old woman may simply state that she went through the menopause at age 45, not mentioning subsequent vaginal bleeding unless specifically asked.

Step 9: Bringing the Interview to a Close

When the student has finished the Systems Review, he should have a reasonably complete history from most patients. It must be recognized, however, that the history will not necessarily be completed in one interview. All the details of the patient's illnesses cannot be obtained in a single session. Additional questions may also be raised in the course of the physical examination, as when the physician discovers the scar of an operation not previously mentioned. If the story is long and complicated, or if the patient is quite ill, the student should be alert to fatigue or discomfort. The interview may need to be interrupted and the patient asked if he would like a brief rest. Again, such sensitivity to the patient's well-being contributes positively to the student-patient relationship and the patient's willingness to cooperate.

As an interview is brought to a close, whether the history is complete or not, it is well to give the patient an opportunity to mention anything else he may have on his mind. This is done by saying "Is there anything else you would like to bring up?" Also, if the student is not clear about a particular area of the history, it may be helpful to recapitulate briefly some of the essential features of the story. In so doing, the interviewer should ask the patient to verify the accuracy of the account: "Now as I understand it, Mr. Jones, your first experience with this pain was early in June, etc." or, one may inquire about a symptom that is still vague: "Now before we finish, let me check to be sure that I am clear about your pain." He then proceeds to relate his understanding of the symptom, inviting the patient to make corrections as he proceeds. Occasionally just as the interview is coming to a close, the patient may introduce some new piece of information as if it were a mere afterthought. The student should be aware that this may reflect concern or embarrassment and that it is important to follow up such information with interest. For instance, at the very end of an interview a patient with a rash may ask "By the way, do you think penicillin could cause this?" Up to this point he had not mentioned that he had recently taken penicillin for the treatment of a urethral discharge.

If in the course of the interview the patient has bared intimate details of a distressing nature or has exposed unpleasant feelings toward family, friends, or doctors, he may later regret that he has said too much. Commonly, he is concerned about the interviewer's opinion of him or that the confidentiality of his communication will be violated. The student may avert such a reaction by reassuring the patient that he understands his feelings and that the information will be handled with professional confidence. In all cases where the patient has been obviously upset during the interview, it is well to return later in the day to see how he is getting along.

When the interview is finished, the patient should be told what is planned next and when. Usually, it is the physical examination.

THE INTERVIEW OF INFORMANTS OTHER THAN THE PATIENT

A physician rarely deals exclusively with the patient. Interested family or friends are almost always present. *It is the student's obligation to meet these persons and to interview, at least briefly, the more important relative or friend.* The reasons for such a meeting are as follows:

1. The student should learn something of the impact of the patient's illness on the family, as well as the influence of the family on the patient's illness.

2. He must learn how to relate to family members so as to be of help to them, as well as enlist their aid for the patient.

3. The visitor serves as a valuable source of additional information and as a check on the reliability of the patient's report of his illness.

4. It gives the student an opportunity to observe directly some aspects of the relationship between the family and the patient.

Arranging the Interview with the Visitor

In general, it is best to interview the patient first before turning to others for information, even when he is limited in his ability to give a history. Only the patient can express his own feelings. His responses in the interview, although incomplete, are most important in understanding him and in diagnosing his problem. Also, unless the situation is urgent or the patient is a young child, it is wiser to interview the patient alone. This affords him privacy and prevents breaks in his flow of thought by a relative who may interrupt in an effort to be helpful. When the patient is interviewed first, the student is also able to learn which visitor is the most appropriate one to interview. To discuss the patient's problems with someone with whom he is on bad terms might jeopardize the student's relationship with his patient. In every case, however, the student should ask the patient's approval to speak with the relative or friend. "I would also like to speak with your wife. Is that all right with you?" If he seems hesitant, the interviewer gives him the opportunity to explain by saying in a questioning tone "If you would rather I'd not. . .?"

Should the patient still remain reluctant, his wish should be respected. Rarely, there are overriding instances when a relative should be seen despite the patient's objection. If so, the matter should be discussed with a staff member.

Most patients readily agree, and indeed, are pleased that the student will meet with the relative. They usually will take it upon themselves to inform the family member. Visitors are also eager to have the opportunity to speak with the staff who are concerned with the patient's care, so usually there is no difficulty in arranging such a meeting.

Conducting the Interview with a Relative or Friend

The meeting should always be in private, although the opportunity should not be overlooked to speak briefly with the patient and visitor together, since this gives some insight into how they interact. To make it quite clear that the meeting is to be more than a hurried casual encounter, both student and visitor should be seated comfortably in a private place before the interview begins.

The student must appreciate that it is an emotionally upsetting experience to have a close relative or friend sick in the hospital. The relative will often need support himself. He welcomes the opportunity to become acquainted with someone involved in the patient's care and appreciates the chance to unburden himself. Indeed, the visitor's distress constitutes an important motivation for his willingness to meet with the student, who should immediately indicate that he is aware of the relative's feelings by asking such questions as "How are *you*?" or "This must be a difficult time for you." These questions allow the visitor to tell about his own distress or ill health as well as about his concerns for the patient or for other members of the family, such as the children. The student must also be alert to the occasions when the relative is not well and is now further troubled by the illness of the patient. This is an especially common situation among elderly couples. The student's willingness to devote some time to listening to the relative's problems not only is helpful to the relative, but also may prevent the visitor from burdening the patient with his own complaints.

Sometimes the visitor begins by asking questions about the patient's condition or about plans for study and treatment. These are best handled by saying that before such questions can be answered, more must be known about the patient; in fact, this is one of the reasons for the meeting. The student may then move to a general question about the patient, such as "Tell me about your husband's illness." *He does not reveal what he has already learned from the patient*, for this may inhibit the informant from giving his own account. Instead, the relative is encouraged to elaborate details, especially in those areas where the patient was vague or where independent corroboration is needed. Often, new perspectives or different facts emerge that require further investigation.

Though usually less detailed, the interview with the visitor follows the same pattern as that with the patient. One identifies the main complaints; delineates the current illness; and explores past illnesses, family health, and relationships, as well as the personal and social history. Since the student already has the bulk of the information, he can more easily follow associations; and with a few well-chosen specific questions, he can verify or round out details already obtained from the patient.

One can sometimes get more information from an informed visitor than from the patient himself, particularly when there are details about which the patient either is unaware or is reluctant to discuss. For example, the patient may not know that his behavior was irrational or that he suffered a convulsion. Or he may minimize, distort, or deny symptoms to completely mislead the student, who may be surprised to learn from the relative how ill the patient has really been. The family member's description of the patient's behavior is especially helpful in the diagnosis of psychosis or depression; indeed, such a diagnosis can be overlooked when information from outside sources is not solicited. The relative's viewpoint is also useful in evaluating how the patient reacts to illness or to hospital procedures, especially when the relative is familiar with how the patient has handled such situations in the past. One may encourage the family members to speak about the patient by asking such questions as "How do you think your wife has been getting along?" "How disabled has she been?" "How has this affected *her*?" or "What sort of a person is your wife?"

Sometimes it is necessary to secure the entire history from a relative. This is particularly important when the patient is critically ill, delirious, demented, or psychotic. Under such conditions, the student carries out the interview in the same manner and detail as he would with the patient himself.

At the end of the interview, the visitor may have more questions. Those that have to do with the patient's condition or plans for treatment are best referred to the physician in charge.

Respecting Confidences When Interviewing Relatives

The confidential nature of some of the communications of the patient, as well as of those of the family, must always be of prime concern. Personal information is not transmitted from one to the other. Above all, the patient is never confronted with conflicting data obtained from another source, unless there is some overriding medical necessity to do so. An example of this would be when the patient withholds an important fact, such as the occurrence of bleeding or a previous venereal infection. If the patient has confided highly personal information concerning the visitor in question, it is especially important to ask his permission before interviewing that particular person and to take special pains to reassure the patient that his confidence will be respected.

The Value of Repeated Contacts with Visitors

Repeated brief contacts with visitors provide an excellent means of following the course of the patient's progress and learning which persons are most concerned about him. Sometimes the visitors will be other than the ones the student expected. For example, a wife's glowing account of her devoted husband may be cast in doubt when it is discovered that he rarely visits, stays briefly, or shows her little attention when visiting. Hence, it is valuable to know who visits and who does not and to observe how the patient relates to his visitor. Significant fluctuations in the patient's hospital course may follow the visits (or the absences) of certain persons. Such observations may prove enlightening in understanding the course of the illness and are important in planning for the patient's care after he leaves the hospital.

Occasionally it is informative to meet together with the patient and with one or more members of the family. This may reveal something of the interactions between family members. Such an interview is usually carried out after the patient has been in the hospital for some time, although very occasionally, an upset patient will insist that the family remain during the initial interview. In this situation, the best approach is to begin with a broad question as "How have things been going?" This is posed in such a way that it is not obviously directed to either the patient or the relative. One can then observe who becomes the spokesman, who contradicts, what exchange develops among the participants, and how they communicate with each other.

Other Sources of Information: Physicians and Hospital Records

On every possible occasion, a student should try to speak with the referring physician or with other staff involved in the care of the patient, such as the social worker or the psychologist. This may be done in person or by telephone. It is particularly important when accurate information is needed about medication, physical findings, and laboratory data. Generally, this is done after the student has interviewed and examined the patient; but in an emergency, or when the patient is incapable of giving a history, the information will be needed promptly. One should always check first with the resident before proceeding.

Bottles of unknown medicines can be identified by a call to the pharmacy that dispensed the drug. From the prescription number, the pharmacist will be able to give the name of the drug, its dose, and directions.

The records of previous admissions to the same hospital or to others should always be carefully reviewed but only after the student has collected his own data. *Reviewing the recorded history in the hospital chart before one interviews the patient usually hinders rather than facilitates the interview.* Only after he has finished his interview and physical examination, and after he has reasoned out his initial diagnostic impression, should the student review the old record. By completing his own study before reviewing the chart, bias is avoided; indeed, the student may come up with a finding or diagnosis unsuspected by others. After reviewing the record, however, he may wish to explore with the patient issues that were raised by previously recorded findings.

SPECIAL TECHNICAL PROBLEMS OF THE INTERVIEW

A number of technical problems may be encountered during the interview. The simplest reflect the insecurity of the student in his newly assigned role, as when the patient consults him about his medical condition or asks personal questions. Others, such as silences, crying, or hostile behavior on the part of the patient, usually stem from the patient's own problems. Clinical experience helps resolve many of the technical difficulties of the interview; however, the student will benefit from a consideration of the following common problems that may occur in any interview:

Questions about the Illness, Procedures, or Treatment

Questions by the patient concerning diagnosis, prognosis, and treatment are best referred to the physician in charge. When such questions are posed early in the interview, the student may point out that not enough is yet known about the patient's problems, which is a reason for his performing an interview and physical examination. If the patient questions him again later, the student should refer him to the physician in charge. "I think it best that you ask Dr. ____________." Sometimes it may even be necessary to ask the patient who he considers his doctor to be. When more than one physician is caring for him, even though all are in complete agreement, it is still best for the physician responsible to do the counseling. Any differences of opinion between doctors may be misinterpreted by patients and lead to anxiety and a breakdown in confidence. On the other hand, the student need not hesitate to answer questions about such matters as ward routine, procedures, or scheduled tests.

Personal Questions

Occasionally, patients will ask the student personal questions. Some may inquire whether a student is married or has children. There is no reason to avoid such questions as long as one does not go beyond the factual data. Other patients will ask questions in a challenging or aggressive manner, often in response to a personal question directed to them. For example, when one inquires about a patient's reaction to a death, he may retort "How would *you* feel?" or "Did *you* ever lose a child, doctor?" Such questions can be answered honestly by saying "I would be very upset" or "No, I haven't." Sometimes the patient asks such a question because he is ashamed or because he feels the interviewer is implying that something was abnormal or unnatural about his reaction. The student's response should emphasize the upsetting nature of such an experience, that people respond differently, and that it will be helpful to know how the patient handled it.

A student may be challenged in a similar way with regard to smoking or drinking, usually because the patient feels accused. "Do *you* smoke, doctor?" is a common rejoinder. A brief honest answer is best, followed by the statement that people's behavior differ and the major concern is with the patient and his health.

Occasionally patients, notably hysterics, manic patients, and a few psychotics, make seductive or even sexual advances. Such behavior must be met in a firm professional manner, and one must avoid getting involved in any type of personal exchange.

Silences

Brief silence on the part of the patient in response to a question should not cause the student to feel uneasy, even though 20 or 30 seconds of silence may seem interminable to the beginner. The pause may reflect the patient's attempt to recall a fact or his indecision as to how he should respond. One can usually tell which is the case from the patient's expression, and the proper behavior is simply to wait expectantly. The student's manner and facial expression should indicate that he expects the patient to continue. If the patient's manner communicates some distress, a response may be facilitated by indicating awareness of his discomfort. This may be done with some remark as "You seem to be troubled," but only after one has waited long enough to see if the patient will resume spontaneously.

A common reason for prolonged or repeated silences is faulty technique on the part of the interviewer. Often, it results from failure to establish a relationship, perhaps because of clumsy handling of the introductory phase, as when some discomfort of the patient is overlooked or ignored. For instance, a patient whose pain or nausea has been passed over is likely to become preoccupied with his distress and may volunteer little information during the interview. Too many specific questions asked too early, especially those permitting only "yes" and "no" answers, or too many interruptions on the part of the interviewer, may give the patient an impression that he is only to answer questions and not to bring up other information. He therefore lapses into the pattern of answering briefly and waiting for the next question. Questions which are too complex may provoke silence simply because the patient does not know how to respond.

Some patients become silent because they have been offended by tactless remarks or a lack of consideration on the part of the student. For example, rushing ahead with a new question before the patient has finished his response may provoke silence; or interrupting when the patient obviously wants to speak of a matter of immediate concern may frustrate him and cause him to become quiet.

When the silences are not due to such technical errors, one may help the patient to resume by such nonspecific comments as "You were telling me about______________" or "Was there anything else?" or "Can you tell me more?" or "Then what?" The interviewer may also simply pick up where he left off and rephrase his last question.

Lack of communication, marked by prolonged silence, may also be a manifestation of organic brain disease, depression, or psychosis.

Crying

It is natural for a student to feel uncomfortable the first few times a patient begins to cry during an interview. Yet, crying is not only a useful clinical sign, it may also afford relief to the patient. Crying usually occurs when the patient is thinking of something that is very distressing to him. This may be the illness or death of a loved one, a threatened loss, or an extremely frustrating situation in his own life. Sometimes, crying is brought on by the patient's concern about his illness and its possible consequence. Whatever the reason, crying is a valuable clinical sign, for it informs the interviewer that the matter under discussion is of grave importance to the patient. The student should wait patiently, allowing the patient to cry and providing a tissue if necessary. By his facial expression, a sympathetic nod, or a kindly remark ("I understand how you feel"), he lets the patient know that he accepts and understands the crying. This enables the patient to relieve his feelings and unburden himself of problems that he may have long wanted to discuss with someone. One does not introduce a new subject until the patient has fully expressed himself and regained control. Such understanding behavior on the student's part goes a long way toward establishing an effective relationship.

At times, it is desirable to invite crying when the patient appears on the verge of tears and is obviously trying to suppress them. A comment, such as "It still makes you feel sad, doesn't it?" lets the patient know that his crying will not meet with disapproval. A student need not worry that he will induce a flood of uncontrollable tears. Usually, the crying subsides in a few minutes and a relieved, often grateful patient is able to resume the thread of his story; and the student will have gained insight into some of the patient's most serious concerns.

Hostility

One may encounter various degrees of hostility from patients during the interview. Some are blatantly hostile, sarcastic, demeaning, or challenging. They may refuse to answer questions, abruptly terminate the interview, or even order the student out of the room. Less overt hostility may be manifested by a curt "I have told all this before" or "My doctor knows all about me; I don't know why I have to tell you." The challenge for the student is to overcome his own natural tendency to become angry. He must try instead to understand why the patient is behaving in such a disagreeable manner. These are always trying situations, especially for a beginning student, but they can be handled appropriately if one is aware of the different situations which may provoke patient anger:

The inconsiderate or angry student.
The patient who is already angry.
The aggressive, pseudoindependent patient.
The demanding, dependent patient.
The paranoid patient.

THE INCONSIDERATE OR ANGRY STUDENT

The first thought should always be whether the student himself has provoked the patient's reaction. Some students always assume that it is the patient's fault and give no consideration to the possibility that their own behavior is responsible. Among the possible ways the student may cause anger are the following:

1. The student may not have adequately introduced himself and made his role clear. The patient may already have been interviewed more than once and may resent being questioned again by someone he believes is not directly concerned with his care. Such a misapprehension on the patient's part is usually corrected when the student explains more fully what his responsibilities are.

2. Interruption of the patient's plan to rest or to visit with family and friends may bring about anger. Also, neglect at the outset to assure his comfort may cause the patient to become increasingly irritated until he explodes in anger at the student, whom he sees as callous and self-centered. The patient uses this means to express himself and bring an unpleasant situation to an end. This predicament may be resolved, even at this point, if the student recognizes the patient's problem and attempts to alleviate it. Sometimes the student has no alternative but to interrupt the interview and start over again at a later time when he can be more attentive to the patient's condition.

3. By failing to pay attention to what the patient has been saying or to keep track of details, the student may repeat the same question or refer to incorrect facts when asking further questions. The patient then finds himself becoming annoyed at the repetition of questions, and may eventually lose patience. Taking adequate notes and allowing more time to formulate the next question usually averts this problem.

4. Questions which are accusatory in tone or inappropriately intrusive may provoke anger. This is most likely to happen when the student fails to follow the patient's associations and asks too many direct questions, such as "Is your marriage happy?" "Were you doing anything that might have caused this?" or "Why didn't you take your medicine like your doctor told you?" The patient may then ask angrily "What does that have to do with my illness?" or refuse to answer. Under such circumstances, the only solution is for the student to recognize his error and adopt a different approach.

5. Failure to appreciate the educational or cultural level of the patient may cause resentment. This is just as likely to occur when a student talks down to an intelligent, well-educated person as when he fails to appreciate the limitations of an uneducated or culturally deprived patient. In both situations the patient feels depreciated. Sometimes such behavior on the part of the student reflects a prejudice; more often it

results from a failure to evaluate the patient's intellectual capability in the introductory phase of the interview.

6. Some patient's reactions reflect the student's personal antipathy, which may be more apparent than he realizes. Everyone has biases, although they are not always acknowledged. The student who finds his patient getting angry will do well to examine his own attitude toward the patient. He may discover that the patient belongs to a category of people whom he dislikes and that he has unwittingly communicated his feeling to the patient, who reacts to his prejudice.

7. Finally, for reasons that have nothing to do with the patient, the student may have approached the interview in an angry frame of mind. He may have been annoyed by a demand of an intern, a criticism by a senior physician, or a letter from home. The patient quickly senses his mood and responds in kind. If the student can recognize his own role in provoking the patient, he should be able to bring himself under control and avoid further difficulty. Sometimes an apology or explanation is indicated.

THE PATIENT WHO IS ALREADY ANGRY

The student may happen to begin the interview at a moment when the patient is still angry about something that has occurred in the hospital or elsewhere. Such anger is readily displaced toward the student, who is a representative of the hospital. The proper response is to hear the patient out, avoid taking sides, and try to be helpful, whether the complaint seems justified or not. It is well to appreciate that the patient can not participate effectively in the interview as long as he is preoccupied with his anger.

THE AGGRESSIVE, PSEUDOINDEPENDENT PATIENT

Some patients act aggressively as a means of dealing with their anxiety or feelings of helplessness. These are people who ordinarily handle their deep-seated fears of passivity by being perpetually active and by vigilantly trying to be in control. To be sick, immobilized, and obliged to submit to the hospital routine is very upsetting. The staff are seen as more threatening than helpful, and hospital procedures which call for passive submission are feared. Such patients struggle to maintain control and overcome these fears, often by acting aggressively toward the staff.

A number of behavioral characteristics forewarn the student that he is dealing with this kind of person. Even when quite ill, the patient is noted to be restless and overactive. He is likely to minimize or deny symptoms, at times passing off major problems as inconsequential. He is quick to tell of his past vigor and to boast of accomplishments. In small but obvious ways, he quickly tries to take control of the situation; for instance, by directing the student where to sit or informing him that he has only a few moments to talk.

The angry outburst may come at any point in the interview, especially when the patient feels his control of the situation is in jeopardy. For example, he may be provoked if the student does not allow him to take the lead or if the student interrupts him or interferes with his way of telling the story. He may become angry when he is pressed for details of symptoms which betray a greater degree of illness than he had heretofore acknowledged. He may cut off the interview when it touches on failures in his work or inadequacies in family relationships.

If the student understands that such outbursts reflect anxiety and the patient's need for control, he will handle such situations in a rational manner. The display of anger should be accepted without retaliation, and the student should attempt to help the patient regain his feeling of being in control of the situation. To accomplish this, the student moves away from the subject matter which provoked the outburst, and he becomes more passive in the interview situation. It may help to explain in very general terms that he needs certain information to be able to understand the problem and do his job. At the same time, the patient is assured that he is not obliged to speak of anything he does not wish to discuss. Such subtle emphasis on how the patient is helping the student in the performance of his duties may serve to reestablish for the patient his much-needed feeling of superiority; for example, one might say "It would help me to understand this if you could spell out what the pain was like." If the patient still demurs, the subject is dropped and the student moves to another area that is more neutral or more conducive to bolstering the patient's self-esteem; for example, one may inquire about a period when he was enjoying good health or having success in his work. If the student succeeds in supporting him in this manner, the patient will often take the initiative by coming back to the subject which led to the outburst.

THE DEMANDING, DEPENDENT PATIENT

An occasional patient voices a never-ending series of angry complaints and demands, making it very difficult to pursue the interview. He sees himself as abused and neglected. These patients are extremely dependent people who feel chronically deprived and are angrily trying to force others to take care of them. They make demands on the student from the moment he arrives; for instance, by asking to have the bed lowered, the shade drawn, or the breakfast tray removed. They may become irritable, angry, and uncooperative when they feel their needs are not being recognized. The student will find that attending to such requests at the beginning of the interview, and even periodically thereafter, will often mitigate the patient's angry demands and lead to a much more productive interview.

THE PARANOID PATIENT

The student may discover that the interview is being interrupted by angry, accusatory questions: "Why do you want to know that?" "Who told you to ask about that?" "Who wants to know that?" "Did my wife put you up to that?" Such questions carry the implication of some devious plan or design that is characteristic of the paranoid patient. The observant student will readily note an underlying quality of suspiciousness in the patient's behavior and an accusatory flavor to his account of the illness. The patient imagines that others are responsible for his plight or have designs against him. The student may be regarded by the patient as someone having a link with these outside forces. Such anger is delusional in origin and is usually beyond appeal to reason. It is wise not to dispute the patient's false ideas, and one should abandon further questioning about the subject which aroused the patient's suspicions.

*****

As with crying, anger does not last indefinitely. The problem may be resolved merely by sitting it out or by coming back to see the patient on some more propitious occasion. It should also be remembered that the patient who does react with anger may later feel sorry. He should be given an opportunity, at that time, to express his feelings of remorse and be reassured that his behavior was understood and accepted as part of the stress of illness. Such a sequence often is the medium whereby an effective relationship becomes possible.

Denial or Withholding

Some patients minimize or completely deny symptoms. This tendency may be a way of averting anxiety, or it may represent a character trait which is the patient's typical manner of dealing with any difficulty. Such patients are not aware of the degree to which they are distorting the facts. Other patients deliberately withhold or distort information about which they are ashamed or afraid. Denial or withholding usually is betrayed by the obvious disparity between the patient's condition and how he reports it. There may be the too hearty, smiling insistence that all is well or that a symptom does not exist. He may dismiss all symptoms by categorizing them as familiar minor disorders, such as "gas," "a little indigestion," "a touch of rheumatism," or "just a virus." Or the patient who is consciously withholding information may respond with repeated flushing, hesitation, revealing gestures, or inappropriate smiling when a sensitive topic is under consideration. As the interviewer recognizes this tendency, he must modify his approach in order to obtain the needed information without provoking anxiety by undermining the patient's defences. This is best done by coming back to the sensitive subject in an indirect manner at a later point in the interview. For example, a patient, fearful of the possibility of heart disease, might refer to his attack of chest pain and shortness of breath as, "just a little gas" or "indigestion." When questioned directly, he may emphatically deny cardiac symptoms. Following the patient's lead, the interviewer should then shift the inquiry to a consideration of digestive symptoms. He asks the patient to tell more about his previous experiences with "gas" or "indigestion" and the circumstances under which they have occurred. Approached from this perspective, the patient may now reveal that in more recent attacks the "gas" sometimes "cuts off my breath" or "squeezes me here" (pointing to his sternum); or that it has come on while playing golf and when he is under emotional pressure. By having the patient describe his daily activities, perhaps later in the interview, one may discover that, over a period of time, he has gradually restricted or eliminated activities because of his symptoms. In this manner, the interviewer succeeds in eliciting the essential details of the history without forcing the patient prematurely to face the possibility of heart disease.

When confronted with this type of patient, it is essential to interview a reliable informant as well. Usually such a person is quite familiar with the patient's propensity to deny or withhold. But with rare exceptions, the patient should not be confronted with the information obtained from an outside source. Occasionally, however, the information is vital and its reliability must be ascertained directly from the patient; for instance, the history of tuberculosis, epilepsy, a psychiatric illness, or of alcohol ingestion. When this is the case, the student will have to explain that the information is necessary if proper treatment is to be instituted, and he must insist on an answer. The probable alcoholic, who admits only to "an occasional beer now and then," may be enticed into a more accurate response when the interviewer suggests a specific amount that might be consumed daily or on weekends. Information which may initially be withheld is often revealed later on a second or third contact, after a relationship of trust has been established.

It should not be forgotten that sometimes the presence of other patients within hearing may be responsible for the patient's withholding information. A later interview in privacy may easily solve this problem.

THE INTERVIEW MODIFIED BY THE PATIENT'S ILLNESS

The student will encounter patients who will be limited in their ability to relate a history because of their underlying illness. In some instances, the acute nature or severity of the patient's illness necessitates an abbreviated interview; in other instances, because of the disease, the patient will be handicapped in telling his story.

The basic outline of the interview is applicable to all situations. There is always an initial introduction, a quick evaluation of the patient's present state, and a series of more detailed inquiries, each proceeding from the more general to the specific. Where it is necessary to modify the interview because of the patient's illness, information must be derived from other sources in order to complete the history. These sources include family, friends, or previous hospital records, as well as the student's subsequent interview of the patient at a more opportune time.

The Acutely Ill Patient

In an acute emergency, the patient's condition demands prompt action. He may be bleeding, in shock, severely dyspneic, in intense pain, or in a psychotic crisis. In such situations, the student must combine the techniques of both the interview and physical examination. Observation of the obvious physical or psychological disturbance is made on approaching the bedside. The student introduces himself and inquires as to the problem. By taking the patient's hand or feeling his pulse, he communicates at once an intent to help as quickly as possible. Except for an occasional psychotic patient, physical contact provides considerable reassurance. At times, it is appropriate to start with a quick examination before questioning him further. Such an approach may reduce the anxiety of a seriously sick person sufficiently enough so that, although previously uncommunicative, he may now be able to respond. As soon as the main area of distress is identified, the student moves quickly by direct questioning to gain the information necessary to determine a course of action. It should be emphasized that, even with the abbreviated work-up of patients in an emergency situation, adherence to the general order of the interview first, followed by the physical examination, will lead to more accuracy; and in the long run will take less time.

The Seriously Ill Patient

In some cases, because of the severity of the illness, the patient cannot be completely interviewed. He may be too weak, too dyspneic, too disorganized, or in too much pain. One must give priority to those aspects of the history which appear most relevant to the immediate situation. Which information is important is not always obvious to the beginner; but in general, the best approach is to explore the first complaints reported by the patient in response to the opening question. If he is having difficulty speaking at any length, more specific questions should be asked sooner than is ordinarily done. It may be necessary to limit oneself to a series of brief interviews for 10 or 15 minutes, distributed over a period of time, rather than to try to get a full history in one or two sessions. For instance, the patient may need more time between bouts of pain or nausea to respond to the questions. In general, by being attentive to the comfort of the patient, the student will succeed ultimately in obtaining an adequate history.

The Delirious or Demented Patient (Organic Brain Disease)[3]

The inability of a patient to report his history in a logical or coherent fashion poses special problems. The interviewer must judge the extent of the patient's deficit, as well as evaluate the reliability of the report. If the patient is capable of providing some of the history, the student adapts his technique so as to make the effort as productive as possible. When the patient appears incapable of giving a reliable history, then a relative or friend must be utilized as the primary source of information. Such serious interference is found in two major groups of disorders: organic brain disease (delirium or dementia) and the functional psychoses, such as schizophrenia, mania and hypomania, or psychotic depression. In practical terms, the student must recognize at the outset that the patient is having difficulty in presenting a coherent story, and an abbreviated mental status examination is carried out to evaluate the nature of the problem. This can easily be done in the framework of the interview.

Patients with organic brain disease have defects in attention, memory, and abstract thinking which make it difficult, if not impossible, to obtain an accurate history. In delirium, the defect is based on a reversible disorder of cerebral metabolism secondary to an inadequate metabolic supply (deficiency of oxygen or glucose), an electrolyte imbalance, or a blocking of the metabolic pathways by endogenous or exogenous toxic substances. In dementia, the defect results from the irreversible

---

[3]Engel, G. L.: Delirium. *In* Freedman, A. M., and Kaplan, H. I., Eds.: Comprehensive Textbook of Psychiatry. Williams & Wilkins Co., Baltimore, 1967, pp. 711-716.

destruction of brain substance, which may develop gradually, as in cerebral atherosclerosis; or abruptly, as with head trauma. Hence, the student should have a high index of suspicion of delirium when he approaches any seriously ill patient, and of dementia when he sees any elderly patient who is sick. Demented patients are especially vulnerable to further metabolic insult, as from hypoxia or drugs; and they will commonly have superimposed the reversible defect of delirium as well.

For practical purposes, the basic psychologic abnormalities are in the cognitive sphere and are the same in delirium and dementia: reduced attention and awareness, defects in recall and recent memory, and reduced ability to think abstractly, as evidenced by difficulty in orientation or in the performance of calculations. Some patients may also exhibit psychotic behavior, with hallucinations, sense deceptions, delusions, or panic. But it is the underlying, usually readily demonstrable, cognitive defect which establishes the diagnosis of delirium or dementia in such patients and differentiates them from those patients with only functional psychoses.

Organic brain disease is first suggested when the patient is noted to be inattentive, unsure of his responses, vague, and inconsistent. Even when answering relatively simple questions, he may appear to be puzzled and to exert an unusual effort. Such a patient responds slowly, hesitantly, with a furrowed brow, and often searches the room as if the answer literally is to be found by looking around for it. He may attempt to deflect the inquiry by humor, sarcasm, or an irritable denial of knowledge. Some patients frankly acknowledge that they are having difficulty in remembering.

When the patient behaves in this way it is wise to interrupt the sequence of the interview and examine the patient's cognitive performance. This is best done by remaining within the general framework of the interview and concentrating on known factual data. Using information in the hospital chart, the student may test the patient's ability to report accurately such items as his home address, his telephone number, the names of relatives, the date of hospital admission, the number of days he has been in the hospital, the present date, and the name of the hospital. One is particularly concerned with the patient's attention, memory, orientation, and ability to calculate. The questions are best posed in the guise of seeking information needed for the record, not in the form of a test. For example, "Which day was it you came here?" "And, let's see, today is the. . .?" "So you have been here how long now?" *The interviewer inquires as though he is the one who is unsure,* and the questions are designed to test orientation for time as well as the ability to perform simple calculations. The latter can easily be evaluated further by having the patient check the ages of relatives against their birth dates. "Your daughter is how old?" "When was she born?" To respond correctly the patient not only must know the current year and remember the birth year, but must also be aware of whether the age reported is consistent with the dates given. By repeating some of the same questions after an interval, one can check on inconsistencies. In so doing, it is often better to behave as if the interviewer himself does not remember, rather than suggesting that it is the patient who does not. "Let's see, how old did you say your daughter is?" In this way, the person with a milder defect is less likely to be offended.

If the patient makes errors in responding to such questions, delirium or dementia is suggested, and a more formal examination of cognitive performance may then be indicated. One may start by asking "Have you been having difficulty in remembering?" coupled with the reassuring comment that this is not uncommon when someone is sick. The patient may then be questioned about his level of education and the type of his employment to give some guide as to his optimal level of intellectual performance. Commensurate with his estimated ability, he may be asked to perform some familiar calculations. A housewife with a grade school education, for example, may be asked to add in her head a small grocery list or to make change. Serial subtractions of 3 or 7 from 100 is a simple and informative technique, but this requires at least a sixth grade education to be reliable. The patient is asked to subtract 3 or 7 from 100 and to continue subtracting until he reaches zero. This tests not only the ability to calculate, but also how well he is able to keep figures in mind without sensory guidance. In the presence of delirium or dementia, the patient exhibits increased effort, takes more time, and makes errors. He may count on his fingers; repeat all the numbers, (e.g., three from 100 is 97, three from 97 is 94, etc.); repeat errors, (e.g., 100, 97, 94, 91, *87*, 84, 81, 77. . .); perseverate, (e.g., 100, 93, 93, 93); lose his place (100, 93, 86, 79, 82, 75); or give some reason not to continue. The student records the length of time taken, the number and kind of errors made, and any pertinent description (e.g., perseveration, concreteness, appeal for outside guidance).

Usually more detailed testing for information, vocabulary, reasoning, and judgment is not needed to establish the diagnosis of organic brain disease, but these procedures are useful when following the course of a delirium.

Patients with defects due to delirium or dementia are not likely to provide a reliable history. The extent of mental limitation should be established early, since it is a waste of time to attempt to pursue a complete interview with such patients. However, the patient who is able to correct errors by exerting more effort can be successfully interviewed. With such a person, the student should word his questions as simply and clearly as possible, give the patient plenty of time to respond, and repeat questions to check the consistency of the responses. Too demanding tasks will increase confusion and provoke fatigue, so it is wise to keep the interview sessions brief. Also, one should not attempt to pursue an interview with a patient who is extremely anxious, hallucinating, experiencing sense deceptions, or who is highly distractible, since this may only serve to upset him further.

The Psychotic Patient

Some patients with psychoses are difficult to interview because they are inarticulate, unresponsive, or silently preoccupied with fantasies, hallucinations, or bodily sensations. Others are difficult because their capacity to relate to others is seriously impaired by disorganized thinking and language, or by behavior which is uncontrolled and bizarre. Yet many clearly psychotic people may give a reasonably reliable and complete history, whether it be of the psychiatric illness or of a concurrent physical illness. As soon as the interviewer suspects that the patient may be psychotic, his approach to the interview is altered in order to incorporate an abbreviated mental status examination. While collecting such factual material as he can, he pays particular attention to the *behavior* of the patient. Is it appropriate and acceptable? Does he display unusual postures, gestures, mannerisms, or inappropriate facial expressions? The *mood* of the patient is noted. Is he in excessively good spirits, profoundly dejected, inappropriately angry, or seductive? His *speech* is evaluated with respect to quality (e. g., tone, loudness, blocking), quantity (e.g., poverty of speech, pressure of speech), and organization (e.g., coherent, circumstantial, flight of ideas, punning). One is alert to *illusions*, where the patient misinterprets sensory data; *delusions*, where he expresses false beliefs; *feelings of persecution, influence, or reference*, where he believes outside forces are affecting him; *hallucinations*, where he sees visions, hears voices, or experiences other false sensations. The patient may have peculiar ideas about his body; for example, that his brain has shriveled up, his nose is deformed, or that one hand is smaller than the other. One also observes how *distractible* the patient is, whether he wanders from the subject or becomes preoccupied and silent.

The patient with a functional psychotic disorder is likely to display abnormalities in many of these areas, yet in contrast to the patient with organic brain disease, he is quite likely to be oriented to date and place, to have intact memory with retention and recall of factual details, and to be capable of performing calculations appropriate to his educational level. Indeed, when discussing matters which are remote from the underlying emotional problems, the patient may be entirely lucid. In practice, this means that the main problem is to deal with the patient's distractibility. The interviewer must repeatedly draw him back to the subject under discussion. With some effort and patience, it will eventually be possible to secure a reasonably complete and reliable account of an organic illness in a psychotic patient.

Psychotic patients who are extremely withdrawn are very difficult to interview. Such patients usually are severely disturbed schizophrenics (catatonic) or are psychotically depressed (retarded). They have great difficulty in making contact with other persons since they are intensely preoccupied with their own morbid thoughts. These patients may be curled up in bed or seated in a slumped position; they may wander distractedly about the room; or may be gesturing, posturing, muttering, and actively hallucinating. Obviously, if such behavior persists for any length of time, a productive interview is out of the question. But some seemingly withdrawn patients will begin to take note of the student and even direct remarks to him if he remains patiently in the room or at the bedside. Very occasionally a patient, who at the outset seemed quite out of contact, may become progressively more responsive; and an interview can proceed, although it is likely to be fragmentary and incomplete. In general, when questions are posed to the more disorganized psychotic patient, he is very likely to stray in his response long before a satisfactory answer can be obtained. Hence, time and persistence are required to piece together the fragments of factual information, and much of the historical information must be gathered from family or friends.

The Depressed Patient

It is important to recognize that many patients with any type of illness may be mildly depressed. This is evident not only from the pessimistic content of their speech, but also is indicated by a lack of spontaneity and a downcast facial expression. The seriously depressed patient, whether psychotic or not, may find it difficult to respond in an interview. He is slowed down and feels burdened or preoccupied. He volunteers little, his responses may be brief, and he does not elaborate. He may complain that he cannot remember or think clearly, although when pressed he is found not to have any significant memory defect. He may express the feeling that it is not worthwhile to report his story, that others are sicker or more in need of attention, and that his own condition is not of sufficient interest to waste the doctor's time. More ominous are expressions of futility, extreme pessimism, self-accusation, and preoccupation with alleged past misdeeds. Thoughts of suicide may be elicited on direct questioning. Psychotically depressed patients ordinarily also complain of poor appetite, constipation, weight loss, and inability to sleep. The presence of depression interferes with interviewing mainly because of the patient's reduced spontaneity and his preoccupation with his own pessimistic thoughts. However, firm but kindly persistence will enable the interviewer to overcome these barriers and to secure an adequate, if not a full account.

Recognition that depression is the cause of difficulty in obtaining a history is of great importance because a suicide risk can exist, and psychiatric consultation may be indicated.

The Mentally Defective Patient

The adult who is mentally defective, unless to an extreme degree, does not manifest a reduced level of awareness or attention. Since he is limited in the ability to learn and perform simple mental operations, he gives the appearance of stupidity or ignorance. This is in contrast to patients with delirium and dementia, whose superficial appearance of stupidity actually is based on a reduced level of attention and a memory deficit. The degree of intellectual retardation of the mentally defective person may be judged by his vocabulary, literacy, and age at the highest grade of schooling. If one is careful to keep inquiry at a level commensurate with the patient's abilities and level of completed education, mental deficiency, unless of extreme degree, usually does not preclude obtaining an adequate history.

The Dysphasic Patient

When a patient has had cerebral injury, such as in a cerebral vascular accident, he may have an expressive aphasia preventing an adequate interview. He may appear totally unresponsive or seem mentally incompetent, but at the same time *can be acutely aware of all conversation around him.* The student must be particularly careful of injudicious comments within the patient's hearing. Such patients may be taught simple signs for "Yes" or "No," enabling some degree of communication. It is also important to recognize that some patients who cannot speak are able to respond in writing.

The Patient Who Is Hard of Hearing

If a patient appears to be hard of hearing, one should always check whether he has a hearing aid available and help him make use of it. If he does not have his hearing aid with him, the assistance of the family or friends should be sought to have it brought to the hospital. The patient who is totally deaf may respond to written questions, or, if able to use sign language, may be able to communicate through an interpreter.

Reference

Engel, G. L.: Delirium. *In* Freedman, A. M., and Kaplan, H. I., Eds.: Comprehensive Textbook of Psychiatry. Williams and Wilkins Co., Baltimore, 1967, pp. 711-716.

Appendix

A VERBATIM INTERVIEW AND CASE WRITE-UP

This section illustrates the course and sequence of an interview and demonstrates how the data so obtained are organized into the case write-up. The physical examination, the diagnosis, and the prognosis are included for completeness and indicate what the examiner considers to be the most important issues of the patient's illness.

The patient is a 52-year-old, married woman, who was admitted to the hospital from another city for an evaluation of symptoms of dyspnea, orthopnea, edema, and rapid heart action. She had recently suffered right-sided weakness. This much was known to the interviewer before he met the patient. The interview was tape recorded and is transcribed verbatim here, except for minor editing to make it more readable and to protect the anonymity of the patient and of her physicians. The interview took approximately one hour. Not all of the necessary information was obtained in the one session, and it would be necessary to see the patient again to completely cover the details.

For the guidance of the reader, a running commentary is printed to the left of the transcript. The commentary highlights the steps of the interview that are outlined in Chapter 3, describes the thought processes of the interviewer, and identifies the principal findings of the patient's history.

Step 1; Introduction
Defining the interviewer's role.

Dr. How do you do, Mrs. Curtis. I'm Dr. Engel. Dr. Morgan has asked me to see you. (extends hand)

Pt. You'll have to take this hand (smiles and offers left hand)

Dr. Uh-huh. Would you sit down here, please? I'm recording this so I don't have to take notes. Do you mind?

Pt. Oh no.

Dr. Good.

Pt. If it all comes out good. (laugh)

Step 2: Defining current status
Interviewer questions "fine."

Dr. How are you feeling?

Pt. Fine! (with emphasis)

Dr. Fine?

Pt. Well, good. (pause) The heart beat is fast, but I'm the same. As long as I don't suffer from it, I don't pay much attention to it. (pause)

Since the patient does not elaborate, the interviewer presses the point.

Dr. When you say fine, what do you mean?

Pt. Well, I don't have anything to complain about. I have no pain. Nothing like that.

Dr. And during the week that you've been here, how have things been?

So far the patient emphasizes improvement and tends to minimize symptoms.

Pt. Oh, fine. I'm getting stronger with the hand every day.

Dr. Your hand is getting stronger?

Pt. Yes.

Dr. Mm-hmmm.

Pt. So yesterday I went to physical therapy. And they showed me some exercises to do, you know, that would make it stronger, so that I can do that myself.

Step 3: The problems leading to hospitalization

Dr. What was the reason for your coming *here* a week ago?

The patient gives a literal response with little clinical information. She continues to avoid speaking of symptoms.

Pt. Well, I was supposed to come here for an operation. I originally was supposed to come sometime in January. The 1st of January my husband took the month off and in December I had the stroke, so I couldn't come. So my physician got in touch with Dr. Y. and told him that he felt perhaps I was over it sufficiently to have the operation. And so Dr. Y. made the appointment and I came.

Chronology.

Dr. When was it originally suggested that you should come here to have an operation?

Pt. In November.

Dr. Before you had the stroke.

Pt. Oh yes. Dr. W. at the clinic at home gave me a thorough going over and he wasn't satisfied.

Dr. This was in . . .?

Pt. November.

Dr. When in November?

Pt. I think it was the 7th?

Dr. The 7th?

Chronology—Election Day as reference.

Pt. It was on Election Day.

Dr. Mm-hmmm.

Pt. And so he consulted Dr. Y, who agreed that I should come back in January to consider having an operation.

Interviewer brings patient back to general question about symptoms.

Dr. Well, when did this all start then?

Pt. Well, during the hot weather, it always bothered me.

Dr. What bothered you?

Her response is vague, so again the interviewer has to press.

Pt. The heat. I can't stand heat, and it's just gotten worse with the years. I was working, you know, as a teller with the First National Bank. And so this first time was in August, on a Friday. I worked under air conditioning. It was, you know, very comfortable. That noon when I went out the door, oh, it was so stifling, and I got a pain in my arm and such pains in my chest! And I couldn't breathe very well. I walked about a block, and I felt so terrible that I turned around and came back to the bank and came in. But then I felt better, so I worked the rest of the day and that night when I went home I said to my little girl that I thought that I'd go see the doctor.

First mention of specific symptoms, pain in arm and chest and dyspnea.

Interviewer indicates interest in child.

Dr. Your little girl is how old?

Pt. Ten years old.

Dr. Ten years old. What is her name?

The patient resumes her account herself.

Irregular heart beat.

"24-hour virus."

Pt. Lois. I went to the doctor and he gave me some quinidine. He said that I apparently had some irregular heart beat, influenced by hot weather. So I took it and I was to go back on Monday. And when I went back Monday, he said that it was fine. So I went back to work that week. The following week the girls weren't feeling too well in the bank. They were having some kind of a virus, like the 24-hour virus or something. And I guess I got it. Three days I had it.

The patient seems reluctant to dwell on symptoms. She hurries through her story. The interviewer tries to encourage her to give more details by bringing her back to the beginning again.

Dr. Let me get this clear in my mind. The preceding period was in August?

Pt. August.

Dr. Did you give me a date, when in August?

Pt. No, I think it was the first part. Say it was the 3rd of August, or something like that.

The interviewer is trying to impress on the patient the importance of dates.

Dr. The first part of August of this past summer, 1967. And you had been working regularly?

Pt. Yes.

Dr. And on that particular day was there some reason why you went out at that point?

Pt. Well, yes, it was my lunch hour.

Patient continues to minimize symptoms. By this time the interviewer knows he will have to press for details if he is to discover the range of the patient's symptoms. Hence he moves into Step 4.

Dr. And how were you feeling that morning?

Pt. I didn't notice anything different. I didn't have any pain or anything.

Step 4: The delineation of present illness

Dr. No pain. You were getting around?

Pt. Yes. In the hot weather I'm used to it. This thing always beats so fast.

Dr. It beats fast in the hot weather?

Pt. Yes.

Dr. So this was something you had noticed prior to that.

The doctors are reported as supporting her use of denial.

Pt. Yes. But I had been to doctors before in the summertime. It seems as though I go to the doctor in the summertime. I tell him that something's wrong with my heart, and the doctor'll say, "No, I can find no defects in the heart." So I go along with it. I think that there's nothing wrong with it.

Dr. Up to that point no one had said there was anything wrong with your heart?

Pt. No.

Dr. How old are you?

Pt. Fifty-two. I'll be 53 on April 11.

Recapitulation to get patient to resume account.

Chronology.

Dr. April 11, uh-huh. So you walked out of the bank and went from the cold to the hot. And what was the first thing wrong you noticed?

Again she is vague and has to be asked.

Pt. It hit my arm. (the patient indicates her left arm)

Dr. What hit your arm?

Pain; location.

Pt. It just pained, my left arm. And, oh, it felt such pains in it, and it felt just like it was beating *so fast.* (puts hand to left upper chest)

Dr. That is where you felt it?

Pt. Yes.

Dr. How did that pain come on?

Pt. It came just like that, it happened.

Dr. All of a sudden.

Pt. Yes, just as I stepped out of the bank, I thought, "Whew, it's so hot, oh boy." It went like that and I didn't know what to do with it, you know. (The patient indicates pain going from chest down arm)

Pain; quality (open-ended question).

Dr. And what kind of pain was it?

Patient has difficulty describing pain.

Pt. Oh, I don't know. It's the kind of pain you have with—sharp pain like, you know . . . well . . . it's something you just can't stand hardly, you know. It's just like that, you know.

Interviewer was going to give her a choice of adjectives, but she selected the first with conviction.

Dr. Was it aching or . . .

Pt. *Yes, yes,* like that. But then it stopped.

Interviewer is echoing her responses as a means of indicating his interest.

Dr. But then it stopped.

Pt. But this didn't stop. (indicates chest)

Dr. The pain in your chest did not stop?

Pt. No.

"This" is vague—must be defined.

Dr. Well, when you say "this," do you mean the rapid heart, too?

Pt. The rapid heart, too. This pain didn't stop immediately. (indicates chest) But then when I was back in the bank, when it got cooler, then it stopped. But the fast heart beat didn't stop.

Pain; duration.

Dr. How long did the pain in your arm last?

Pt. Oh, I went from the bank down into the next block before it stopped.

Dr. Walking slowly?

Pain: aggravating factor

Pt. Yes, I had to walk very slow because it was so painful.

Pain; location (open-ended question).

Dr. Now where in the arm did you feel it?

Pt. It seems as if it was everywhere. (laugh)

Dr. As if it was the whole arm?

Pt. Yes.

Dr. Did it seem to be inside or on the outside of the arm?

Pt. Well, I don't remember that. It just hurt so bad that I don't remember . . .

Pain; location (specific question).

Dr. Did it go into your hand?

Pt. No, I don't think so. . . I don't know.

Interviewer invites patient to speak of the other symptoms: palpitation and dyspnea.

Dr. You don't remember that. And then you came back in, and you noticed that your heart was beating fast. You also mentioned that you were short of breath.

Pt. Yes.

Dyspnea; quantity.

Dr. How short of breath were you?

Pt. Well, I sort of had to take a deep breath in order to draw it, you know.

Pain; duration.

Dr. Uh-huh. So then you came back into the bank and you say your arm pain disappeared. How soon did the chest pain disappear?

Pt. Oh, it was . . . about 20 minutes.

Dr. About 20 minutes.

Pt. Mm-hmmm.

Palpitation; duration.

Dr. And what about the pounding of the heart?

Pt. No, that didn't let up. I went home, and then I went to the doctor's.

Noting the tendency to minimize, the interviewer wants to explore the fact that the patient stayed at work after her attack.

Dr. Uh-huh. But you continued to work.

Pt. Yeah, yes . . . for a few days.

Dr. No, I mean that day.

Pt. Oh yeah. I worked until 5 o'clock.

Dr. You were going out for your lunch, but you didn't have lunch?

Pt. I didn't eat.

Dr. You just came back to the bank and went back to your window?

Pt. Mm-hmmm.

Dr. How come?

The patient is revealing a personality style, to ignore or minimize disability. The interviewer knows this will have to be taken into account if he is to obtain a full history

Pt. I don't know. The doctor had told me there was nothing wrong with my heart. So I thought, well, there's nothing wrong with it, so I continued to work. I didn't know what else it could be.

Dr. Is that like you, just to go on about your business if you can?

Pt. Yes.

Interviewer recapitulates to encourage the patient to resume her account. In so doing he also emphasizes his interest in details.

Dr. Mm-hmmm. So you went back to your job without your lunch. The arm pain subsided, then the chest pain; but your heart continued to beat fast. You went home at five and told your little girl that you were going to the doctor's.

Pt. Mm-hmmm.

Dr. And he gave you the quinidine.

Pt. Mm-hmmm.

Dr. Can you pick up the story from there?

The patient skips the weekend.

Pt. Then Monday I went back to him, as he asked me to.

The interviewer brings her back.

Dr. Well, how were you over the weekend?

Pt. Fine! (said with vigor) The quinidine made it calm down.

Chronology.

Dr. The quinidine calmed it down how soon?

Pt. Oh . . . I don't remember how long. It was fine when I went to the doctor's on Monday.

The interviewer doubts the patient's "fine!"

Dr. Well, how did you spend the weekend, do you recall?

Pt. It was an ordinary weekend. Of course, I couldn't go out. On Saturdays I always do, but that day I just couldn't. Sunday was quiet.

Setting.

Dr. Who was at home that weekend?

Pt. My husband and my son and my daughter.

Brief exploration of family.

Dr. You have two children?
Pt. I have three.
Dr. Three.
Pt. One is married. One's 16 and one is 22 and one is 10.
Dr. The 22-year-old is a boy or a girl?
Pt. Boy.
Dr. What is his name?
Pt. Bob.
Dr. He's married?
Pt. Mm-hmmm.
Dr. And lives where?
Pt. In the same town.
Dr. What is the 16-year-old's name?
Pt. Mark.
Dr. So there were the four of you at home, you, the two younger children and your husband.
Pt. Mm-hmmm.

Resume account of illness.

Dr. And it was an ordinary weekend.
Pt. Mm-hmmm.
Dr. And Monday you went back to work?
Pt. Mm-hmmm. But I didn't feel so good.
Dr. What was the trouble?

Patient again bypasses details of symptoms.

Pt. Well, I was apparently coming down with the virus. And so I worked all that Monday. Tuesday morning I went to work, but I only worked an hour and I felt sort of sick.

Interviewer insists.

Dr. Well, how did you feel, coming down with the virus?

Patient again skips details.

Pt. I had cold chills and such fever. First you have a chill and you'd be so cold. So I went upstairs and I told the personnel manager that I wanted to go home, and he said all right. So I was sick Tuesday . . . all of the rest of the week. And so the next Monday I went back to work.

Interviewer presses for more details.

Dr. You had cold feelings . . .
Pt. Mm-hmmm. And, oh, I sweated so, I dripped sweat, ooooh!

Open-ended question.

Dr. And what else did you notice that week?
Pt. That's the type of thing that I had.

Finally asks specific questions when patient does not elaborate.

Dr. Aching?
Pt. No.
Dr. Sick to your stomach?
Pt. No.
Dr. Diarrhea? (patient shakes head "No"). Were you short of breath?
Pt. Yes.

Open-ended question.

Dr. Tell me about being short of breath.
Pt. Well, I was just awfully short of breath and . . . (pause)

Dyspnea; quantity.

Dr. How short? What could you do?
Pt. I didn't do anything. I stayed in bed and finally got over it, at least I thought I was over it and then Monday . . .

Patient evades discussion of dyspnea; interviewer insists.

Dr. I want to know a little bit more about the shortness of breath in that week. How much could you do without getting short of breath?

Pt. Well, very little. (hesitantly)

Dr. Very little?

Pt. Very little.

Dr. Did you do the kitchen work, for example?

Pt. Very little. (laugh)

Dr. In what position did you rest in bed? Could you lie flat?

Pt. No, I had two pillows.

Orthopnea.

Dr. Two pillows. How long have you had two pillows?

Pt. Oh. . .quite a while. Especially in the hot weather.

Dr. Was this a matter of years or . . .

For the first time she indicates a longer duration. The interviewer notes this in his mind to come back to later. He continues with the current episode.

Pt. Oh yes, well, I would say a couple of years.

Dr. A couple of years?

Pt. Yes.

Dr. Was there any change in that week in terms of the number of pillows?

Pt. Well, I don't know if there was any change or not, but it felt more comfortable to sleep with the two pillows.

Dr. Did you wake up at night feeling short of breath?

Pt. Yes, in hot weather.

Dr. Did the shortness of breath wake you up?

Nocturnal dyspnea.

Pt. Yes.

Dr. And what would you do when you woke up?

Pt. Nothing. I'd just wake up and be there. There's a small window behind my bed, and my husband put a screen in and it would open and I used to have it hooked back.

Interviewer checks associated symptoms.

Dr. Did you have any wheezing in your chest?

Pt. No.

Dr. Or coughing at night?

Pt. No.

Dr. I gather this shortness of breath is something that goes back some time.

Since the patient has mentioned dyspnea, orthopnea, palpitation, and chest pain, the interviewer now inquires directly about other cardiac symptoms. Edema.

Pt. Yes, a couple of years.

Dr. A couple of years. Did you notice any swelling of your ankles?

Pt. Yes. By 6 o'clock at night my ankles would look like, yeoww. (laugh) They'd get so big!

Dr. How far back does that go?

Pt. Well . . . in the hot weather it was worse. Well, it's been increasing, you know.

Dr. Since?

Now acknowledges 3 or 4 years of symptoms.

Pt. Oh . . . I would say about 3 or 4 years.

Dr. Three or 4 years.

Pt. It would come off and on. But then this past year by the time summer came, every night.

Edema, aggravating and alleviating factors.

Dr. Every night. So there was a change this past summer in that you noticed that by evening your feet would be swollen every night.

Pt. Yes.

Dr. And by morning, how would they be?

Pt. By morning it would be gone.

Interviewer resumes thread of present illness.

Dr. Be gone. Now let's come back to after this flu episode.

Pt. Well, after the flu episode I went back to the bank to work on Monday, and on Tuesday I was to go down to the . . . doctor and see if this was taking effect. I didn't think it was taking effect because I could feel it beating so fast.

Tachycardia; chronology.

Dr. When did you first begin to feel this beating again?

Pt. Well, I felt it all weekend.

Dr. But it had gone the first week?

Pt. Yes, before then. So I went down to him and said, "I don't think the medicine has taken effect." Well, he didn't know, of course, that I had the virus, so he asked me a little bit about it and he took my blood pressure and my pulse and he said, "Where is your husband?" And I said, "He's home." And he said, "Well, go to the hospital." So I went up to the hospital and he put me in Intensive Care. He thought I had a heart attack.

Date, first hospitalization.

Dr. On what date was that?

Pt. I think it was the 15th or 16th . . .

Doctor's name.

Dr. Of August. Who is your doctor?

Pt. Dr. Jones. And then he called in Dr. Watson, who is a heart specialist, and he gave me a cardiogram. And then they decided I didn't have a heart attack. They didn't know what it was. And so after Dr. Watson had given me two or three goings over, he decided that I had leakage or something like that.

Dr. And is this the first time that anyone had ever mentioned leakage or a murmur or anything of that sort?

Pt. Yes.

Chronology.

Dr. So you were in the hospital how long?

Pt. I was in 2 weeks, until September 3.

Course.

Dr. And during the time you were in the hospital, how were you?

Pt. Oh, it was the same, the rapid heart beat and so forth, that I had at home.

Dr. You continued to have the rapid heart beat.

Pt. And then I went home and I had a rapid heart beat and I had one digitalis pill—a digoxin?

Dr. When did you begin the digoxin?

Pt. In the hospital. I was also on blood thinners when I was in the hospital, but then they took me off it. And I didn't take any more. I just had the one digoxin. And when I went home Dr. Jones found out that my heart was beating too fast, so he went to Dr. Watson, who said I should take two digoxins.

Dr. At the time that you left the hosptial, what recommendation was made?

Pt. Well, it was that I should go home and just do light housework and see how I got along.

Dr. Was there any discussion of surgery at that time?

Pt. Yes, he said I would possibly have closed heart surgery but he said, "We'll let this go for the time being." But by November, when I didn't get any better, he called Dr. Y. and arranged for me to come up here in January.

Interviewer explores reaction to prospect of surgery.

Dr. Uh-huh. What was your feeling about that proposal at that time?

Patient minimizes.

Pt. I didn't care.

Interviewer presses.

Dr. You didn't care. What do you mean, you didn't care?

Pt. Well, if I'm gonna get better, I would have to have an operation.

Open-ended question.

Dr. And what was your life like during those weeks at home?

Pt. Well, I didn't go out, except once a week. I used to go to the grocery store with my husband, but that's all. And I got along all right. I knitted, oh, I don't know, about that high pile of sweaters and that sort of thing. I knitted right along and did light housework. And December 11, boom, I had the stroke!

Stroke, December 11, 1967.

Open-ended question.

Dr. Tell me about that.

Pt. Well, it was 11 o'clock at night, which was a little late for me to be up, but I was making a carton to put on the door to fit the newspaper in. 'Cause I didn't want the boys to throw it in the snow and get it damp. And so I thought I would put a little fancy paper on it so it would look better, because I was using a milk carton. And I put the staples on the outside. Sometimes the staple gun sticks, so I was trying to fix that stapler so it would not stick. And I went to put in a second staple and my fingers felt all tingly, you know. (massages right hand) I thought, "Gee, that's funny." I didn't know why they should go to sleep when I was using it. So I just put it on my lap like that, and, gee, it felt, you know, it felt terrible! And then I felt as though I was drooling. So my son had gone to bed and for some reason he got up to get a drink of water and he said, "Mother, what are you doing?" and he looked at me. He said I looked so funny. So he ran to the telephone and called my father—my husband. "You better come home. Mother's sick."

Slip of the tongue.

Interviewer notes husband was not home at 11 p.m. and wonders why.

Dr. Where was your husband?

Pt. He was at the New York Central Railroad. He's a car inspector.

Dr. He works at night?

Pt. Well, he works different hours. And so my husband came right home. And in the meantime my son said, "You'd better get on the bed." And I didn't know the leg had gone. So I got up and I fell on the floor. It was just too much, you know. So he picked me up. I don't remember him picking me up but they did, and took me into the bedroom and then I . . .

Dr. You don't remember them picking you up?

Pt. No, but I became conscious of the fact that I was on the bed and I kept going in and out, you know. And they said both sides of my neck swelled way out.

Establishing duration of unconsciousness.

Dr. Uh-huh. So you were unconscious just between the time that you got up and fell down and the time they picked you . . .

Pt. Well, I kept going unconscious. I remember going to the hospital. . .

Dr. You remember falling?

Pt. Yes.

Dr. Now who carried you in?

Pt. My husband, I guess.

Dr. Your son had called your husband. And had he already come before you had fallen?

Pt. I don't know. He came home within 10 minutes.

Dr. Within 10 minutes.

Pt. Uh-huh.

Dr. So you were unconscious for not more than 10 minutes.

Pt. That's right.

Dr. Then when you were on the bed you were sort of in and out of consciousness.

Pt. Yes. It was the same thing in the hospital. I remember going to the hospital, but I don't remember taking my clothes off.

Dr. Did you have trouble speaking?

Aphasia.

Pt. Yes.

Dr. What was the trouble?

Pt. Well, I couldn't make anybody understand. (laugh) Nobody could understand me for about 3 days.

Dr. Would the words form in your own mind?

Pt. Yes.

Dr. Did you know what you wanted to say?

Pt. Yes.

Open-ended question.

Dr. Well, how were these 3 days for you?

Pt. Well, time went by so fast that I couldn't believe that 3 days had gone by. And then time kept going and things kept coming better and I moved my leg in the bed. So after 6 days I left Intensive Care.

Details of the course.

Dr. When did you first begin to speak understandably?

Pt. The third day.

Dr. By the third day.

Pt. Yeah.

Dr. Uh-huh. And your leg was the first to come back?

Pt. Yeah.

Dr. First your leg improved, then your speech?

Pt. Uh-huh. They didn't all improve, you know, but I could make my husband understand what I wanted.

Dr. How were you feeling during those days in Intensive Care?

Pt. All right.

Interviewer checks cardiac status.

Dr. You felt all right? What about your heart circulation? Were you aware of anything?

Pt. Well, I didn't suffer any pain or anything.

Dr. Were you short of breath?

Pt. No.

Dr. Were you having a rapid heart?

Pt. Well, as I say, I'm so used to having a rapid heart that I don't pay any attention to it.

Dr. So then you were in the hospital for how long?

Pt. Let's see, 4½ weeks.

Interviewer inquires about experience of being away from home during holidays, since this is often upsetting to patients.

Dr. That brings us up to January—you must have been there over Christmas and New Years.

Pt. Oh yeah, all the holidays.

Dr. All the holidays?

Pt. Oh yes! I nearly had a fit to have to stay in the hospital over New Years and Christmas.

Dr. Why?

Pt. Oh, I wanted to be home, you know, with my children, but then I got sick.

Dr. You nearly had a fit?

Pt. Well, I felt terrible, you know. I—well, I cried. (laugh)

Dr. You cried. That's understandable.

Pt. But I got over it.

Patient acknowledges upset but minimizes it.

Dr. You felt sad and unhappy at that point?

Pt. Sad for myself, probably.

Recapitulation.

Dr. Uh-huh. Let me go back now. The stroke was December 11, and you had been discharged from the hospital in September?

Pt. September 3, I think it was.

Dr. So it was about a 3-month period that you were home.

Pt. Yeah.

Open-ended question to elicit more information about illness since September.

Dr. And you told us that you took it easy and you knitted that pile of sweaters and things. What *were* these 3 months like for you?

Pt. Well, at first I thought it was kind of boring, but then I put up with it because I thought, "Well, it has to be done. And after I have the heart surgery, well, I'll be all right."

Dr. You felt you'll be all right.

Pt. So I just took it.

Dr. What restricted your activity? Was it what the doctor said you could do or was it . . .?

Pt. The doctor said what I could do.

Dr. You did what the doctor said.

Pt. Yes.

With indication that patient has been an active person, interviewer wonders how she adjusts to enforced inactivity.

Dr. And I have the impression that ordinarily you're a fairly active person.

Pt. *Yes*, very much so! (with emphasis)

Dr. Very much so. Can you say a little bit more about that?

Pt. Well, I'm a person who walks a great deal. I'd walk from here to Timbuktu. (laugh) I like to walk.

Dr. You like to walk.

Patient emphasizes activity.

Pt. I mean I go to church every Sunday, and I always walk. I do *all* my grocery shopping, I do *all* my other shopping downtown and everything. And last September I never went downtown or went any place, but I thought, "Well, I want to go but I'll do something else."

Evaluation of disability by exploring daily activity.

Dr. And the two children were at home?

Pt. Yeah.

Dr. And how much of the housework did you do?

Pt. Well, I just did—running dustmops and that sort of thing. When it came to mopping or something, then my husband would do that.

Dr. Your husband would do that.

Pt. Mm-hmmm.

Dr. Did you try to?

Pt. No.

Dr. Why not?

Pt. My doctor said not to. (laugh)

Dr. The doctor said not to. Do you have stairs in your house?

Pt. Yeah.

Dr. Did you climb stairs?

Pt. The doctor said not to go up and down stairs any more than I could help and so I didn't.

Dr. And when you did go upstairs . . .

Dyspnea, one flight of stairs.

Pt. It would make me short of breath, even if I went up slowly.

Resume chronologic account.

Dr. It would make you short of breath. Okay, then let's come back now to the date of your discharge from the hospital, which would have been January . . .

Pt. Oh, I don't know, about the 17th.

Second hospitalization: 12/11/67-1/17/68.

Dr. In other words you were in the hospital from the 11th of December to the 17th of January?

Pt. Yeah.

Dr. And what did you do after the 17th?

Pt. Nothing, I can't use that right hand, you see. Although, I couldn't even do this much when I was home. (demonstrates that she can raise right hand almost to chin) So my husband got all the meals and gardening.

Dr. You're right-handed.

Pt. Yes.

Interviewer returns to earlier piece of information.

Dr. You mentioned earlier that your husband was going to take off the month of January.

Pt. Yep! He did!

Dr. He did. He had already planned that.

Pt. Yeah.

Dr. Uh-huh. When had the admission to this hospital been scheduled for?

Pt. In January.

Dr. No definite date, but sometime in January.

	Pt. Yeah.
Course after discharge from hospital.	*Dr.* Uh-huh. Then you were home from the 17th until this past Friday, the 26th. Were you in bed or in a chair or walking around?
Fatigue.	*Pt.* I got up every morning and during the day I would lay down twice, because if I didn't, I'd be so shook up, you know, so tired.
Clarify term, "shook up."	*Dr.* Shook up—what does shook up mean?
	Pt. Well, you just can't go on. (laugh)
	Dr. Uh-huh. Fatigue.
	Pt. Yeah.
Fatigue; location, quality.	*Dr.* How do you feel the fatigue?
	Pt. Well, it wouldn't be so much in my chest. I was just all in, you know.
	Dr. All in.
	Pt. Yeah.
As a point of reference interviewer comments on how patient walked in.	*Dr.* Uh-huh. Well, you walked fairly well when you came in the room here this morning.
	Pt. Yes, that has improved, too.
	Dr. That has improved since you are here?
	Pt. Yeah.
Interviewer explores patient's reaction to stroke.	*Dr.* Mm-hmmm. What is your understanding of the stroke?
	Pt. An artery or something burst back there on this side, I guess, and it affected this side. (indicates left side of head)
	Dr. Have you had any knowledge or experience with stroke?
	Pt. Yeah, well, I have had from other people, you know.
	Dr. Who?
	Pt. My aunt.
Family history of strokes: aunt, father	*Dr.* Your aunt?
	Pt. Mm-hmmm. But she's still living; she's 82.
	Dr. Uh-huh. When did she have her stroke?
	Pt. A couple of years ago. And I took care of my father, and my father had a stroke.
	Dr. Your father had a stroke, too?
	Pt. Yes.
	Dr. When was that?
	Pt. Oh . . . let's see, he was 74. It was about 16, 17 years ago. And I took care of him. So I knew about it then too.
	Dr. Mm-hmmm. How long did you take care of him?
	Pt. Oh, from March until the last of August.
	Dr. Till August.
	Pt. Mm-hmmm.
Interviewer takes opportunity to explore early relationships and Family Health while getting details of father's stroke.	*Dr.* He lived with you?
	Pt. No, I lived with him.
	Dr. You were married at that time.
	Pt. Yeah, oh yeah.
	Dr. So you and your family lived. . .
	Pt. With my father, uh-huh.

Dr. With your father. Uh-huh. And on which side was he paralyzed?
Pt. This side. (indicates left)
Dr. The left side.
Pt. His stroke was in his leg mostly.
Dr. More in his leg.
Pt. It was just terrible.
Dr. Terrible, how do you mean?
Pt. And in his voice.
Dr. Voice.
Pt. He couldn't get up. He used to try to get up to go to the bathroom, and he couldn't stand up at all.
Dr. This was quite a problem in nursing him.
Pt. Yeah.

The closeness of the relationship to the father prompts the interviewer to explore this further.

Dr. How did you happen to be the one who took care of him?

Patient second of five children.

Family always depended on her.

Pt. Well (laugh), I'm next to the oldest one of five children, and for some reason my father, my people have always depended on me. My brothers and sisters always depended on me and so I've always taken care of them, help 'em get whatever they want.
Dr. Are you the oldest girl?
Pt. No. There's another older girl, but she is . . . well . . . let's say immature. She's married, but she just isn't mature.
Dr. Uh-huh. How do you mean she's not mature?

Older sister mentally defective.

Pt. Well, the doctors have said that as she grows older, she will grow more immature. At times she has the maturity of a 15-year-old girl.
Dr. Mm-hmmm. How much older than you is she?
Pt. Two years.
Dr. Two years. So did you have to help her out when you were young?
Pt. Yeah. (laugh)
Dr. But she did marry.
Pt. Yeah.
Dr. Had children?

Nephew has Down's Disease, institutionalized.

Pt. She had two. And one boy was Mongolian. He's still living, but he's in a home.
Dr. Uh-huh. And the other boy?
Pt. The other boy's all right.

Interviewer now returns to explore the period prior to August, 1967.

Dr. Well now, let me go back to before this past August. You say for a couple of summers you had noticed this intolerance of the hot weather, that your heart beat fast, and that you had been getting short of breath. Can you tell me now how far back this goes, that you were having any trouble at all?
Pt. Well . . . (sigh) I don't know. It's . . .well, it could be 4 or 5 years.
Dr. It might be 4 or 5 years.
Pt. It came gradually . . .

Chronology.

Dr. And what was the first thing you noticed, do you think?

Pt. You mean this past summer?

Dr. No, going back 4 or 5 years.

Tachycardia.

Pt. Well . . . It was just the heart beat got rapid.

Dr. A rapid heart beat.

Dependent edema.

Pt. And the swelling of the legs.

Dr. Under what circumstances?

Sudden increase in edema 2 years ago.

Pt. A couple of years ago I had . . . an accumulation of water. I put on 13 pounds in a couple of days.

Dr. Two years ago?

Pt. Yeah.

Dr. When?

Pt. In the summer.

Checking dates.

Dr. In the summer. Which summer?

Swelling of abdomen.

Pt. 1966, I think. In June or July; I don't remember. And I went to the doctor's. I got up one morning and I couldn't even put a belt on. So I thought, "My God!" I didn't know what had happened to me. So I went down to the doctor and he said, "Well, I'll give you some water pills and I'll give you a couple of days to take that off and if you don't, we'll send you to the hospital," And gee, I went right at it and I took it right off. It never happened again.

Response to diuretic.

Dr. You urinated it.

Pt. I had to stay right near the bathroom. (laugh)

Dr. Were your legs swollen at that time, too?

Pt. Everything.

Dr. Were you short of breath?

Pt. Well, I don't remember. I suppose I was. It was in the summertime.

Dr. You emphasize the summertime. In the wintertime . . .

Relation of symptoms to hot weather.

Pt. The wintertime I don't pay any attention to it, because in the wintertime I like the cold weather. You can breathe so much easier, and you don't have the hard time to do anything. But the doctors have always said there's no trouble, so I forget about it.

Interviewer challenges patient's minimizing.

Dr. You say you forgot about it. I'm not sure what that means.

Pt. Well, I just didn't pay any attention to it.

Dr. You mean you had the symptoms, but you didn't pay any attention to them?

Pt. Yeah.

Dr. So you might have a fast heart rate in the winter as well as the summer . . .

Pt. Yeah.

Dr. . . . and your feet might get swollen in the winter.

Pt. They don't get swollen *so bad*, up until the last winter. They didn't swell near as much.

Dr. But they *did* swell some?

Pt. Some, yes.

Interviewer tries to establish onset.

Dr. When was the first time that you ever noted any swelling of your feet?

Pt. Oh . . . gee, I don't know. It's . . . a long time. I just can't tell you how long it's been. It's been a long time, because it comes gradually, you know.

Dr. Uh-huh. And would the swelling always go down at night again?

Pt. Yes.

Dr. So you're simply not sure when, but it's a number of years, maybe 4, 5 years that you've had the swelling, more in the summer than in the winter, but you *do* have it in the winter but it just doesn't trouble you as much.

Pt. Yeah.

Dr. And so, too, with the fast heart rate. You have that in the winter, but it doesn't bother you so much.

Pt. Mm-hmmm.

Interviewer tries to clarify whether true orthopnea or paroxysmal nocturnal dyspnea has occurred.

Dr. And for how long is it that you've been sleeping on two pillows?

Pt. A couple of years.

Dr. What does a couple mean?

Pt. Oh, two, I guess.

Dr. What started that? Why did you start moving to two pillows?

Pt. Well, because I thought I could breathe easier.

Dr. You thought you could breathe easier. And did you?

Pt. I thought I could.

Dr. Uh-huh. Did it ever occur at any time that you awakened at night extremely short of breath and had to sit up or stand up?

Pt. No, I didn't ever do that.

Dr. You mentioned your husband fixing the little window.

Pt. Mm-hmmm.

Dr. I don't have clear what that was for.

Pt. Well, it's a dormer window, a small window. So he opened that and I slept right beside that, you see.

Dr. So that you would have more air?

Pt. Yeah.

Dr. I see.

Patient emphasizes association between summer and dyspnea.

Pt. It's the summertime that it seems that something cuts off the air. (laugh)

Step 5: Past Health
Because of the patient's reluctance to speak of illness, the interviewer focuses on her work and life activities, anticipating that these may have been interrupted by illness.

Dr. Mm-hmm. During this 4- or 5-year period, up to this summer, aside from what you've told me, what was your health like?

Pt. All right.

Dr. All right? No other illnesses?

Pt. Nothing has been wrong.

Dr. No other illnesses, no hospitalizations . . .

Pt. No.

Dr. And during that time, have you been working?

Pt. Yes.

Dr. How long have you been working at the bank?

Pt. A year.

Dr. Hmmm. Had you worked before that?

Pt. No. I worked before I had the children, for 7 years or so. I worked at a paper company.

Dr. I see.

First pregnancy—baby died of heart disease.

Pt. And then I had a baby, but it lived only 6 hours because he had a . . . well they said a bad heart.

Dr. This was the first child?

Patient avoids mentioning symptoms.

Pt. Yeah. And then I went back to work after that and I worked for about . . . 2 months. And then I thought I had heart trouble. So I went to the doctor . . .

Interviewer asks.

Dr. What trouble did you have?

She still avoids.

Pt. The doctor said he thought I had thyroid trouble. So I went into the hospital and had a basal metabolism test, and it turned out negative.

Chronology.

Dr. When was this?

1943, 25 years ago.

Pt. Oh . . . let's see . . . 25 years ago.

Dr. Twenty-five years ago. And this was a few months after the birth . . .

First mention of possible valvular defect.

Pt. Yeah. And then after they said that was negative, the doctor said, "Well, go to Dr. E., he's a heart specialist." So I went and he said, "Well, the only thing I can say is that you've got a little scar tissue in there because of having rheumatic fever when you were 8 years old." So I didn't go back to him. It didn't seem necessary. I only came back to him for a corrective, you know, to see if it was all right. So I went back to him for a few times and he says, "Well, it's all right." And the last time I went he said, "Well, gee, I can't find anything wrong; you're all right."

Still no mention of symptoms.

Interviewer repeats question.

Dr. What symptoms were you having that led you to see the doctor?

Pt. I was having rapid heart beat, and I was short of breath.

Setting.

Dr. Rapid heart and you were short of breath. You noticed the shortness of breath under what circumstances?

Pt. Oh . . .well, I don't know. It was so short, you know, all the time. When I was young like that and I thought, well, maybe that I had heart trouble. But the doctor . . .

Dr. I didn't follow that.

Pt. He—I thought that I had heart trouble because I had such short breath.

Duration.

Dr. How long had you been having short breath?

Pt. Well, since I had that baby.

Establishing time of onset.

Dr. Were you short of breath during the pregnancy?

Pt. No.

Dr. Not during the pregnancy.

Pt. I didn't think so.

Dr. Uh-huh.

Pt. And I told the doctor that I thought I had heart trouble and he said, no, that he thought that I had a little scar tissue.

Dr. Were you short of breath in bed?

Pt. No . . . well, I don't remember all that.

Dr. You don't remember.

Dyspnea; quality, "frequent sighing."

Pt. You know, it's been so long and all, but I remember that at the time I had frequent sighing.

Dr. Frequent sighing?

Pt. Yes. I felt I could hardly get a long breath. You just want to get a long breath like that and that's what really made me wonder if I did have heart trouble.

Dr. Was that what you mean by shortness of breath at that time?

Pt. Yeah.

Dr. The sighing?

Pt. Yeah.

Dyspnea; setting.

Dr. And did this come on at any particular times?

Pt. No . . .

Dr. It could be while you were sitting as well as standing or walking?

Pt. Mm-hmm. Yeah.

Dyspnea; quality.

Dr. You just feel you have to get in a deep breath.

Pt. Mm-hmmm.

Dyspnea; chronologic association with death of baby with heart defect.

Dr. And you say the baby, they said, had heart trouble.

Pt. Yeah.

Interviewer explores patient's reaction to the loss of baby.

Second pregnancy, 1946.

Dr. How did it affect you, to have lost that first child?

Pt. Well, it was something that I had planned on and I, you know, I felt bad that I had lost it. So then 3 days—3 years later I had a son. And my children are all right.

Dr. Did you cry?

Pt. Yeah.

Dr. You felt sad? (patient nods head) How long did it take before you got over it?

Pt. Well . . . probably a year.

Dr. Probably a year. Were you trying to get pregnant in the interim?

Pt. No.

Dr. You were not.

Pt. No, I was told not to.

Dr. You were told not to? Why?

Pt. Well, I don't know. The doctor that delivered the baby said I should wait a year and a half, at least, before I'd even attempt to.

Dr. Did he say why?

Pt. No.

Dr. And to this day you don't know why.

Pt. No.

Dr. And then after a year and a half did you try?

Pt. No, my husband wasn't too much in favor of my having another one so soon.

Dr. Why not?

Pt. Because he didn't want me to go through it again.

Dr. He didn't want you to go through what again?

First acknowledgment of symptoms during pregnancy. Nausea, vomiting.

Pt. Well, every time I get pregnant I get very sick. For 9 months I'm throwing up and everything. After a while I convinced him that I probably wouldn't have it again. So I had another one. But I was just as sick!

Open-ended question.

Dr. Uh-huh. Throwing up and what else?

Epistaxes.

Pt. And I had terrible nosebleeds. At the time I threw up, I'd lean over the toilet like this and I—once something happened to my eye and it all turned black. I don't know what it was.

Check chronology.

Dr. This was the first pregnancy?

Pt. No, the second.

Since the patient has opened the subject, interviewer will pursue obstetrical history.

Dr. The second one.

Pt. And I had to go to the doctor frequently every week or so and then the baby was all right when it was born.

Interviewer explores specific symptoms during pregnancies.

Dr. What happened to your weight during these pregnancies? Did you gain or lose or . . .?

Pt. That first one, I didn't gain too much.

Dr. Didn't gain too much.

Edema.

Pt. No. The second one, I gained. Oh, I had an awful lot of water.

Dr. The second one you gained a great deal.

Pt. Oh yes.

Edema; quantity.

Dr. How much? Do you remember?

Third pregnancy, 1951.

Pt. Oh, about 20 pounds. My legs swelled so—and my feet—that I couldn't get anything but bedroom slippers on. The next, that was 5½ years later, I was so sick in the third month that the doctor put me in the hospital and I had glucose, I guess. And then when I came out, the same thing happened all over again. So he said, "Well, the only thing that I can do is take the baby." But I didn't want him to do that so I said I would get through it somehow. So I went along and I got through it all right but I didn't lose the swelling of the legs there, oh, it was a long time. It was all of—he was born in July. It was October or something like that.

Edema; duration.

Dr. This would be 16 years ago.

Pt. Yes.

Specific symptoms: dyspnea.

Dr. Were you short of breath during that pregnancy?

Pt. Yeah.

Dr. How about the first two pregnancies? Were you short of breath?

Pt. I don't remember whether I was short of breath or not.

Dr. But you remember well that you were short of breath with the third one.

Pt. Yeah, uh-huh.

Dr. Did you have high blood pressure with any of these?

Pt. No, he said it was low blood pressure.

Low blood pressure.

Dr. Low blood pressure.

Headache, vomiting.

Pt. It would hurt the top of my head, you know, when I would throw up and I thought I had high blood pressure. And so I spoke to him about it; he said, "No," he said, "it's low blood pressure."

Dr. Did he ever say you had anything in your urine?

Pt. He never took any.

Asks about fourth pregnancy.

Dr. Now what about the last pregnancy, 10 years ago?

Bleeding.

Pt. I thought I had lost it. At 2 months I think it was, I had a hemorrhage and I had big, big blood clots, *big* blood clots. The doctor came and said, "Well, I think you've passed it." So after about 3 or 4 days in bed he said, "No, you're still pregnant." So I went home and I was home another month, then I had another hemorrhage. And he said, "Well, we'll go to the hospital again." So he thought I'd lost it again. So he examined me and I was still pregnant. I went home after a week and I stayed home until the baby was born.

Dr. Did you gain as much weight this fourth time?

Edema.

Pt. No, I didn't, but my legs swelled.

Dr. Your legs did swell.

Pt. Yeah.

Dr. Were you short of breath this time?

Dyspnea.

Pt. A little.

Dr. A little bit.

Edema, duration.

Pt. But then afterwards I stayed swollen around my middle and I still had swelling in my legs until quite a while afterwards.

Dr. Both legs.

Pt. Mm-hmmm.

Interviewer wonders about thrombophlebitis to account for edema of legs.

Dr. In any of the four pregnancies, was there any difference in the size of the legs?

Pt. The third one, it was worse.

Dr. No, I mean was there any difference in swelling between the left leg and the right leg.

Pt. No, I don't think so.

Dr. Were your calves ever tender?

Pt. They always have been.

Dr. They always have been.

Pt. If you pinch 'em like that.

Dr. Was the fourth pregnancy planned?

Pt. No. (laugh) We were kind of surprised.

Dr. Uh-huh. You were already 41, 42.

Pt. Yes, 42.

Fourth pregnancy unplanned. Interviewer inquires about patient's reaction.

Dr. Uh-huh. How did you feel about it at the time?

Pt. Well, I wasn't planning on it and I was a little bit . . . skeptical whether I'd carry it through. And my husband felt terrible about it. He thought it . . . was gonna be kind of hard on me. But I said, "We'll let be what's to be, so don't get upset about it."

Resume survey of Past Health.

Dr. Any other illnesses during these years?

Pt. No.

Dr. Have you been in the hospital other than the pregnancies and the times that you told me?

Tonsillectomy, age 9.	*Pt.* I had my tonsils out when I was about nine.
	Dr. Uh-huh. Any injuries?
	Pt. No.
	Dr. Or accidents?
	Pt. No.
Interviewer brings patient back to "rheumatic fever" at age eight.	*Dr.* Tell me about the rheumatic fever when you were eight.
	Pt. Yeah, since I've grown up they call it rheumatic fever, but of course they didn't call it that then. They just said rheumatism because they didn't have the know-how then. I didn't go to school all one winter, my legs swelled so. And I couldn't get my shoes on. And I don't remember what went on there, but I know that I went to get the tonsils out because I don't remember whether I had sore throats or not, but they said that as a result of this I should have my tonsils out.
Swelling of legs.	
Edema, location.	*Dr.* And your legs swelled where?
	Pt. From the ankles up to the knees.
	Dr. The whole leg was swollen.
	Pt. Yeah.
	Dr. Both legs.
	Pt. Mm-hmmm.
Inquires about symptoms of acute rheumatic fever.	*Dr.* Was it sensitive? Were your joints sore or painful?
	Pt. I don't remember.
	Dr. You don't remember that. Did you have swelling of any other parts of your body?
	Pt. No, no.
Checks other features of edema.	*Dr.* Was your face puffy when you woke up in the morning?
	Pt. I don't remember.
	Dr. Did you have rheumatism anywhere else?
	Pt. No.
	Dr. Do you remember whether you had fever?
	Pt. No, I don't remember.
Childhood illnesses.	*Dr.* Any other illnesses in childhood?
	Pt. No.
	Dr. Did you have St. Vitus Dance . . .
	Pt. No.
	Dr. Did you have sore throats when you were young?
	Pt. If I did have, I don't remember.
	Dr. You don't remember. Scarlet fever?
	Pt. No.
	Dr. Diphtheria?
	Pt. No.
	Dr. Do you remember any other childhood illnesses?
	Pt. No. I remember I had mumps and measles, that sort of thing, but they were light, you know.
Not satisfied with story of "rheumatic fever," interviewer returns to it.	*Dr.* You say you had to stay home from school that whole winter.
	Pt. Yes.
	Dr. Why?
	Pt. Because I couldn't get my shoes on, just bedroom slippers. So I had to stay home.

Dr. And did you stay in bed or around the house?
Pt. Well, no, I stayed around the house, you know.

Step 6: Family Health

Dr. Uh-huh. Where were you living at that time?
Pt. In Geneva.
Dr. You lived in Geneva all your life?
Pt. Yeah.
Dr. And your family comes from Geneva?
Pt. Mm-hmmm, mm-hmmm.

Interviewer begins with known information—father's death.

Dr. Your father, you say, was 74 when he died, 17 years ago?
Pt. Yeah.

Father's work.

Dr. What did your father do?
Pt. He was truckdriver for Roberts Hardware.
Dr. And he worked until when?
Pt. He worked right up until March, until he had his stroke.

Father's health.

Dr. What was his health like?
Pt. He was wonderful.
Dr. Always in good health?
Pt. Yes.
Dr. And do you know what was the cause of his death?
Pt. The stroke . . . only.
Dr. The stroke, that's all?
Pt. Mm-hmmm.
Dr. And when he was young, what did he do?
Pt. He was an auto mechanic.

Mother.

Dr. And your mother?

Died at 49.

Pt. My mother was very sickly. My mother died at 49.
Dr. Forty-nine. You were how old?
Pt. Oh, let's see, I was 23, 24. Oh no, let me see, 27.
Dr. Twenty-seven.
Pt. Yes.

Interviewer recognizes mother died same year as did first baby.

Dr. Twenty-five years ago.
Pt. Yes.
Dr. When was your mother's death in relationship to your first pregnancy?
Pt. Oh, it was about . . . I became pregnant just a few months before she died.
Dr. She died before you delivered?
Pt. Yeah.

Two losses, mother and baby.

Dr. So you had two losses that year, didn't you, the baby and your mother.
Pt. Yeah.
Dr. What was the cause of her death?

Mother's health: leukemia, hysterectomy, cholecystectomy, appendectomy, chronically sick.

Pt. She had *so many* sicknesses! She finally died of cancer of the bloodstream. But before that she had had a hysterectomy and she had had her appendix out and then she had gallbladder trouble. Just sickness all the time.
Dr. One thing after another.
Pt. Yeah.

Interviewer links mother's chronic ill health and patient's role as the helper.

Dr. So was this the reason why you were the one who was taking care of everybody?
Pt. Yeah.

Mother's symptoms.

Dr. Did she have shortness of breath?

Pt. I don't remember. I don't believe so.

Dr. Or weakness?

Pt. She took some kind of digitalis or something; I don't know what it was now.

Dr. Did you help take care of your mother?

Pt. Yeah.

Inquires how mother's death affected her.

Dr. How did her death affect you?

Pt. Well, we felt very sad when she died, because, well, she's my mother.

Dr. Do you think about her still?

Pt. Not . . . I don't think . . . it don't bother me.

Siblings.

Begins with sister already mentioned: Bessie.

Dr. Now the five of you, the oldest one is a girl.

Pt. Bessie.

Dr. And you told me about her. Bessie is married and she lives where?

Pt. In Geneva.

Dr. And the one after you is . . . ?

Brother: John.

Pt. That's John.

Dr. John.

Heart attack, March, 1961 or 1962.

Pt. And he has a heart attack—a heart condition. He had pneumonia 6–7 years ago, the 16th of March.

Dr. The 16th of March.

Pt. Mm-hmmm, and as a result of the pneumonia, he got a heart attack. I don't know why, but he has blood clots, so many of them that he has to take blood thinner. And he has to go every week for a blood test. He doesn't work.

Work.

Dr. Has he worked since then?

Pt. No.

Dr. What did he do?

Pt. He worked in a machine shop. He was a grinder, I guess you'd call it.

Age.

Dr. How old is he now?

Pt. He's 51.

Dr. He's a year younger than you.

Pt. Yeah.

Marital status.

Dr. And he's married?

Pt. Mm-hmmm. He has a little girl.

Dr. Little girl.

Pt. Eleven years old.

Dr. Uh-huh.

Sister: Geraldine.

Pt. And then I have a sister, Geraldine, that's in good health. She had a hysterectomy, but she's fine.

Dr. She's how old?

Pt. She's 47.

Marital Status.

Dr. She's married?

Pt. Mm-hmmm. She has five children.

Dr. Five children.

Brother committed suicide, March, 1967. Patient breaks down.

Pt. Mm-hmmm. I have another—I did have another brother, and he committed suicide last March. He had a lot of trouble. He had a lung out and . . . well, that was just all. (crying)

Interviewer allows patient to cry; expresses understanding. She then spontaneously gives more details.

Dr. It's hard. (pause) Still affects you deeply, doesn't it? (patient crying for about 2 minutes) It must have been quite a shock at the time.

Pt. A terrible shock.

Dr. Mm-hmmm.

Patient uses present tense, "lives."

Pt. He lives in Westford, Virginia. And he had come to see us the last of March because he said he hadn't seen John, who was my brother who had the heart attack, 'cause he hadn't seen him in such a long time and he wasn't too well at the time. And he says, "Well, I think I'll come over and see him while he's alive." But he never did.

Dr. Did you have warning of this, or . . . ?

Pt. No.

Dr. Was he married?

Pt. Yeah, he has three children.

Dr. Three children. How old was he?

Pt. He would be 45 in April.

Dr. Uh-huh, he was the baby. What was his name?

Pt. Merlin. He was full of spirit, lots of good laughs, you know, and everything.

Dr. Any understanding of what happened?

Pt. No. You see, I live here and he lived down there. He used to call me about once a month. And that month he didn't make that call to me and then I got a telephone call. (pause, sniff) I didn't go down for the funeral because I said that I couldn't go down and meet his wife. You know, we never got a chance to go down there. He used to come home every summer and so I said to myself, "Well, I can't do him good anyway. Because if I got down there I would be *sick* and . . .

Interviewer responds to patient's comment that she would get "sick" if she went to funeral.

Dr. You would be *sick*?

Pt. Yeah. I was afraid I would be sick, so I would rather stay home.

Dr. When you say "be sick," what did you have in mind?

Pt. I don't know. I don't know.

Dr. You just had the feeling that you would be sick.

Pt. Yeah.

Dr. So you did not go to the funeral.

Pt. I did not go.

Dr. Mm-hmmm. How do you feel about that now?

Pt. I still wouldn't go.

Dr. You still feel that was the right thing to do.

Pt. Mm-hmmm.

Inquiry into grief reaction.

Dr. You cried at the time?

Pt. Yeah.

Dr. And you still cry.

Pt. Well, occasionally. (smiles weakly)

Interviewer comments on evidence of close relation with brother.

Dr. So it's almost a year now, isn't it? The first year is always the most difficult. I have the feeling that you and your brother were quite close.

Pt. Oh yes! I always – he's my little brother and whenever he'd get in trouble and would want to talk to somebody, he always called me.

Inquires as to patient's health at time of brother's death.

Dr. Always came to you, uh-huh. How was your health at that time?

Pt. I was good. I was working for an insurance company at the time.

Dr. This was March of '67?

Pt. Yeah, I told you that I was working for a year for the bank. I should have told you I worked for an insurance company before that and then I began work for the bank last April. And the insurance company had about as good as folded.

Further query about brother's death.

Dr. How did your brother commit suicide? Do you know?

Pt. He shot himself.

Dr. Shot himself. (pause) What was his work?

Pt. He was in marketing with the GE company.

Dr. I see. Had he been depressed?

Pt. I don't know.

Dr. Had he ever been depressed?

Pt. Not that I know of.

Dr. But you say he had had problems.

Pt. Yes, he had had with his lung.

Dr. With his lung.

Brother's chronic lung disease.

Pt. I would say about 12 years ago he had a lung removed because – it wasn't a lung cancer. They said it was something that had made it porous. So they took off everything up to about here (indicates midchest), and they sewed it up and left it like that. And so he came home and only about 2 weeks later it started a whistling sound. It was terrible! So then they said, "You'll have to go back to the hospital." The thing had leaked into the cavity, and they put this big tube in his back and he lay for 8 weeks and then they pulled that out of him. And gosh, it was terrible. And I went to see him almost every day.

Dr. He lived in Geneva at the time?

Pt. Uh-huh. But he got over it. He was fine.

Dr. What symptoms did he have?

Pt. Mostly he coughed up a lot, sometimes he had blood in it. And he'd get pneumonia.

Dr. He was married at that time?

Pt. Yeah.

Dr. But he had other troubles more recently?

Pt. No. Well, just that. I don't know now. I heard the doctor had told him that his other lung was starting to get that *same* disease. The doctor told me at the time that if that ever happened again he would suffocate. And so if the doctor had told *him* that, perhaps that's why he committed suicide.

Dr. He didn't leave a note?

Pt. No. Not that I know of.

Dr. Not that you know of. Are you in contact with your sister-in-law?

Pt. Yeah.

Dr. How has she been?

Pt. She's been fine.

Dr. She's been all right.

Pt. They've got a beautiful home down there, three teen-age daughters.

Resume Family History—marriage.

Dr. Now, you've been married how long?

Pt. It'll be 30 years in November.

Dr. Thirty years, and your husband is how old?

Husband.

Pt. He's 50.

Dr. Fifty.

Pt. He'll be 51 . . .

Dr. Uh-huh, he's just a little younger than you are.

Pt. Yeah, two years.

Husband's health.

Dr. Two years younger. And how has he been?

Pt. Fine.

Dr. He works for the railroad?

Pt. Uh-huh.

Work.

Dr. And has for how long?

Pt. All the time.

Dr. And what is his job?

Pt. He's a car inspector.

Dr. That's a big New York Central yard there, isn't it?

Pt. Yeah. Well, It isn't so big any more since they're merging, you know, so what they're going to do now, we don't know.

Dr. Is his job in any jeopardy?

Pt. No.

Dr. Being a car inspector means what?

Pt. Checking the air brakes and all that sort of thing.

Dr. Uh-huh. So he's had long years with New York Central.

Pt. Uh-huh. It takes another year, February I think it is, a year from this February, he will have 30 years in under the present pension system.

Dr. And you say he's been well?

Pt. Yes.

Husband's reaction to patient's illness.

Dr. How is he taking your sickness?

Pt. He's doing very well. (laugh)

Dr. He's doing well.

Pt. He's a good housekeeper. (laugh) And he's taking care of the children.

Children.

Dr. And the children, how have they been?

Pt. Fine.

Lois.

Dr. Lois?

Pt. She's just fine.

Dr. And she is in school?

Pt. Mm-hmmm.

Dr. And has she had any illnesses?

Pt. No.

Mark.

Dr. Any problems? (shakes her head, no) And how has Mark been?

Pt. Oh, he's a big guy. He's about 6 foot now and he's never had any problems.

Dr. He's in high school?

Pt. Yeah, He's a junior; he'll be a senior.

Dr. And how is he doing?

Pt. Fine.

Dr. Fine. His grades are good?

Pt. Oh, good.

Dr. Any problems?

Pt. No.

Dr. His health has been good?

Pt. Fine.

Dr. Uh-huh. And what's he heading for?

Pt. Well, he doesn't know. First he's going to be a teacher and then he's going to be something else, but the most he's talked about is being a teacher.

Dr. Then he'll probably go on to college, you think?

Pt. I think so.

Robert.

Dr. And your oldest boy, Robert, is 22.

Pt. Yeah.

Dr. Is he married?

Navy 4 years ago.

Pt. He's married. He's very well. He joined the Navy Reserve when he was 17, and he's been away in the service after he graduated high school for 2 years and then came home and he got married before he finished the service.

Dr. When did he marry?

Married 2 years ago; baby, 7 months old.

Pt. He's been married 2 years. He was 20 when he got married. And now they have a little—7 months old now.

Dr. Seven months old, uh-huh. And his wife?

Pt. She's well.

Dr. Uh-huh.

Pt. And the baby's cute.

Dr. Your first grandchild!

Pt. Yes. (smile)

Dr. And his wife's name is what?

Pt. Judy, she was a little Italian girl.

Patient indicates poor relationship with daughter-in-law.

Dr. Uh-huh. And do you see much of them?

Pt. Not too much. (smiles)

Interviewer inquires.

Dr. Uh-huh. How come?

Patient opposed marriage.

Pt. Well, (laugh) when he wanted to get married, I didn't want him to get married until he was 21. But he insisted no matter what I said to him. And so finally I said, "Well, as long as you want to get married, get married. I'll sign for you."

Dr. Uh-huh.

Pt. So his father and I signed for him. But his wife was a little bit—she's very, well . . . Italian people are like that. They're very much for their own family, for the sisters and brothers and father and mother, you know. And, well . . . she's always nice enough to us when Bobby would bring her over. We're always nice to her and she's nice to him—to John (sigh). But, I don't know, there's something strange about it. And to this day I don't think she's ever come into the house without Bobby, you know.

Dr. Never by herself?

Pt. No.

Dr. So it's not a very warm relationship for you.

Pt. No.

Dr. Mm-hmmm. And what was their marriage date?

Married May 9, 1966.

Pt. May 9, 1966.

Dr. The spring before last.

Grandson, June 27, 1967.

Pt. Yeah. That would be it. And they've got a little baby 7 months old. He was 7 months old the 27th of January.

Dr. So he was born in June of '67.

Pt. Yeah.

Interviewer wonders about religious differences.

Dr. What is your religious background?

Pt. I'm Protestant.

Dr. You're Protestant. And Judy, I assume, is Catholic?

Slip of the tongue.

Pt. Yeah. But that doesn't make any difference, you know. My father—my husband is Catholic.

Dr. He is Catholic.

Pt. Mm-hmmm.

Dr. So that wasn't an issue.

Pt. No, no. I think probably because I didn't want him to be married when he was only 20 because he had no job. He had nothing and so I wanted him to wait until he had more to offer. But this girl is—she's very nice. She took it as if we don't like her.

Dr. How old is she?

Pt. She's two years older than he is.

Dr. Two years older than he. What is he doing now?

Pt. He's working for B. Company.

Dr. Doing what?

Pt. He's got a good job. He's some kind of inspector. It isn't anything he wants to do all his life, you know.

Interviewer indicates he appreciates the problem.

Dr. This is kind of a problem mothers have with children, isn't it?

Patient minimizes.

Pt. Yeah. Well, for me, I don't let it bother me.

Dr. You don't let it bother you.

Pt. No.

Return to Past Health.

Dr. Now I think I have a pretty good picture of what your health has been. Any other illnesses that . . .

Pt. No.

Dr. You say you have had no operations.

Pt. No.

Allergies, sensitivities.

Dr. Do you have any allergies?

Pt. No.

Medication.

Dr. Or sensitivities, hay fever, asthma? (shakes head, no) Are you taking any other medication now?

Digitalis.

Pt. I'm taking some digitalis. I can't tell you how much because one day I take three and yesterday I took one. Today I'll take two or something. I don't know.

Dr. When did you start the digitalis?

Pt. When I first entered the hospital in Geneva.

Dr. What else do you take?

Pt. Blood thinner.

Dr. Which blood thinner?

Pt. I don't know.

Coumadin.

Dr. Coumadin?

Pt. Yes, coumadin!

Dr. Coumadin. And how much do you take?

Pt. One five a day.

Dr. One five a day. And how often do you get your blood tested?

Pt. Every day. (laugh) Every day I've had my blood tested every day for 5 weeks in the hospital and for—that week I was home I went every other day to the hospital and I've had it every day, sometimes three times a day since I've been here.

Dr. Uh-huh. Any other medications?

Pt. No.

Asks about other cardiac measures.

Dr. Are you on any diuretics . . .

Pt. No.

Dr. . . . or anything to make you urinate?

Pt. No.

Dr. Have you been at any time since this started?

Pt. No.

Diet.

Dr. Are you on any diet?

Pt. Well, salt free.

Dr. You've been on a salt-free diet since . . . ?

Pt. Since I was in the hospital in September.

Dr. How low is the diet?

Pt. Well, I guess it's pretty rigid.

Dr. Do you take milk?

Pt. No.

Dr. Do you add salt to the cooking?

Pt. No.

Quinidine.

Dr. What about the quinidine? I gather the only time you had it was when you had the pain and palpitations, last August.

Pt. Yeah.

Dr. How many pills a day did the doctor give you then?

Pt. It was about three a day.

Dr. Three a day.

Pt. Yeah.

Dr. And so you took that for a total of how long?

Pt. Well, I was only I would say . . . oh about a week and a half.

Effect of quinidine.

Dr. About a week and a half. During that time did the palpitations change particularly? You said it was better on the first weekend, I remember, but . . .

Pt. It just seemed much better.

Dr. In what way?

Pt. Well, it seemed to calm down.

Checking detail of palpitations overlooked earlier.

Dr. When these palpitations first started, were they regular or irregular?

Pt. Oh . . .

Dr. Were they very fast like that or . . . jumping around?

Pt. I would say that it was going irregular.

Dr. And as you went out the bank door, did the palpitations start gradually or suddenly?

Pt. Well, suddenly.

Dr. And you had had palpitations before in the summer and . . .

Pt. Yeah.

Dr. Was this different in any way than what you had before? Did it feel different in any way?

Pt. Yes, I could feel it a lot worse.

Dr. In what way?

Pt. Oh, it felt as though it was more than usual, you know, it was unusual.

Dr. More severe?

Pt. Yeah.

Step 8: Systems Review *(Patient has already provided sufficient information about development and current situation so that Step 7 is unnecessary.)*

Dr. Do you have headaches at all?

Pt. No.

Dr. Have you ever had any injuries to your head?

Pt. No.

Dr. You've been wearing glasses for how long?

Pt. Oh, I've worn glasses since I was about 20.

Dr. Mm-hmmm. Are you nearsighted or far . . .

Pt. Nearsighted.

Dr. Nearsighted. Any problems with your eyes other . . .

Pt. No.

Dr. Blurring vision or double vision?

More information about stroke.

Right homonymous scotomata.

Pt. During the stroke I had things wavering in front of my eye like that, you know, if I look up to the light. At first I thought it was something with my glasses, you know.

Dr. On the right side.

Pt. Yeah, the right side. And so I took off my glasses, and gee, it still kept coming so I thought, "Gee, I wonder if it could have been from the stroke?" So I spoke to the doctor and he said, "Sure."

Dr. Uh-huh. Did you notice it when your eyes were closed?

Pt. Yeah. You know, you close 'em like that and the eyelids would flutter so. (laugh)

Dr. Did you have any difficulty closing your eyes with the stroke?

Pt. No, no.

Dr. Any other problems with your eyes?

Pt. No.

Dr. Any blurring of vision after that?

Pt. No.

Dr. Do you get colds, often?

Pt. No, I don't.
Dr. Any trouble with your nose?
Pt. No.
Dr. You mentioned nosebleeds with pregnancy.
Pt. I had that just once during pregnancy.
Dr. The first pregnancy.
Pt. The second one.
Dr. Second pregnancy.
Pt. I had such nosebleeds.
Dr. Any other time?
Pt. No.
Dr. Never again.
Pt. No.
Dr. How about your teeth?

The patient's reference to "so darn much medicine" should have been followed up.

Pt. Well, my teeth aren't too good because I had taken so darn much medicine when I was a kid. This is—these four teeth are capped. And I've only got one, two, four back teeth.
Dr. Any infections?
Pt. No.
Dr. Abscesses, toothaches?
Pt. Every time I had a tooth pulled it was abscessed. I guess it was abscessed. Yeah, I think it was abscessed. . .I kept enough of all these back teeth.
Dr. How about your hearing?
Pt. No trouble.
Dr. No trouble with your ears, earaches? Ringing of the ears?
Pt. No.
Dr. Sore throats?
Pt. No.
Dr. Did you ever have any difficulty swallowing?
Pt. No.
Dr. And did you ever have pneumonia?
Pt. No.
Dr. Ever coughed up blood?
Pt. Well, I have during the pregnancies.

Hemoptysis during pregnancies.

Dr. During the pregnancies. Was that in relationship to the nosebleed or was it separate?
Pt. No, separate.
Dr. So you coughed up blood. Which pregnancy?
Pt. All of 'em.
Dr. All of them. Just during the pregnancy?
Pt. Yeah.
Dr. And what was it like? When you coughed up blood?
Pt. It was just . . . right in with the sputum, and so forth, you know.
Dr. You were coughing at the time?
Pt. I always started coughing before I vomited.
Dr. And how many times did this happen that you coughed up blood?
Pt. Well, I don't know how many times.
Dr. Two or three . . .

Pt. Yeah . . .

Dr. . . . or . . . or a dozen?

Pt. Not every time.

Dr. Did you have x-rays for this?

Pt. No.

Dr. Or a bronchoscope; anybody ever look down your throat?

Pt. No.

Dr. Would it be a little bit of blood or a lot?

Pt. Oh, just a little bit.

Dr. Did you notice shortness of breath?

Pt. I don't remember.

Dr. I neglected to go back to one thing, the pain in the chest that you had . . .

Pt. In August?

Dr. In August. Had you had pain in your chest at any other times?

Pt. No.

Dr. Ever have any pleurisy?

Pt. No.

Dr. Mm-hmmm. What about your digestion?

Convulsions to age 14.

Pt. Well, they always said that I had nervous indigestion. From the time I was born until I was about 14, I had convulsions. I would have something to eat mostly at night and if it was heavy then I would get sleepy and I'd go and lay down, and I'd have a convulsion. So for years—I can't tell you how many it was—I didn't eat supper. I ate the same thing I ate for breakfast.

Open-ended question.

Dr. What were these convulsions like?

Pt. Well, I can only tell you my mother said that she didn't ever know whether I was gonna live or die, your eyes go back and you just—you don't . . .

Specific questions.

Dr. Did you bite your tongue?

Pt. Yeah, well, no, no. I would not. Some people jerk all over, you know, but I didn't.

Dr. You didn't. Did you ever wet yourself?

Pt. No.

Dr. Your eyes would roll back and you would pass out?

Pt. Just pass out.

Dr. And you don't remember anything.

Pt. No. And when I come to, my mother and father would be rubbing my arms and legs.

Dr. You say this disappeared when you were 14.

Pt. Yeah. At 14 I had about three of them in one night and that was the end of it.

Dr. And they gave you medicine for that?

Pt. Yeah. First one and then another. I've taken more medicine than could be lined up on this floor.

Dr. Do you know the names of any of those medicines?

Pt. The only thing I can remember is . . . luminal.

Dr. Luminal? Dilantin ever?

Pt. I don't know. That's the only thing that—that's the only thing that sticks with me.

Dr. Bromides? Do you remember that?

Pt. No, I don't remember anything. But I do remember that my mother used to say that she never was satisfied. At first they gave me medicine for epileptic fits. And my mother said that was not the epileptic fits that I had because she had seen epileptic fits. And so she wouldn't give me any medicine. And then, oh, I've taken so much medicine and then so many doctors.

Dr. What did your mother think the fits were?

Pt. She didn't know what they were. She wouldn't have anybody say they were epileptic fits.

No family history of epilepsy.

Dr. Any history of epilepsy in the family?

Pt. No, no.

Dr. Now any gas or indigestion, or nausea and vomiting, other than during pregnancy?

Pt. No.

Dr. Ever have yellow jaundice?

Pt. No.

Dr. What about your bowels?

Pt. Oh, they're good.

Dr. No trouble there. Have diarrhea?

Pt. No.

Dr. Blood. Hemorrhoids?

Pt. I have hemorrhoids.

Dr. What trouble do they give you?

Pt. They don't give me any problem at all now. But the last time I had trouble I think I had a blood clot. I didn't know what it was. Oh, it was terrible. I tried to doctor myself and I thought it would go away and all of a sudden I saw blood, a great deal of blood from . . .

Dr. When was this?

Pt. This was about five years ago. And so I went to the doctor and he said, "Well, it's a good thing that it happened. Your problem is over with because it had broken." I—he said, "I would have had to lance it." So I haven't had any trouble since.

Dr. And what about your urination?

Pt. Good.

Dr. No trouble. Do you get up at night?

Pt. No.

Dr. Never have. Any pain in your back ever?

Pt. No.

Dr. Ever see blood?

Pt. No.

Dr. No history of kidney trouble?

Pt. No.

Dr. Bed wetting when you were young?

Pt. No.

Dr. High blood pressure?

Pt. No.

Dr. Never had high blood pressure.

Pt. No.

Dr. And what about your menstrual periods?

Pt. I'm still having them.

Dr. Have they been regular?

Menorrhagia.

Pt. Yes. In fact, the first part of January I had a menstruation period, and it just kept carrying on and on and so the doctor gave me a D and C.

Dr. When did you have the D and C?

D and C January 11, 1968.

Pt. About the . . . oh, I'd say about the 11th or 12th, something like that.

Dr. About three weeks ago.

Pt. Yeah.

Dr. And what did they tell you about the D and C?

Pt. They said it was all right.

Dr. It's okay. Have you had any problems with your menstruation over the years?

Menorrhagia, September, 1967.

Pt. Well, in September. It just got awful; it got out of control. I just walked across the floor and I had to clean up the floor afterwards. And so I called the doctor and he said, "Well, if you can come down, you better come down." And so I went down there and he gave me a shot.

Dr. This was after you were here?

Pt. Yes.

Dr. Uh-huh. So you have had several prolonged or profuse periods since September. When did your periods start? How old were you?

Pt. Fourteen.

Menarche, 14.

Dr. You were 14.

Pt. Mm-hmmm.

Interviewer notes menarche and cessation of convulsions both at 14.

Dr. How about the relationship between the start of your periods and your convulsions?

Pt. That's one thing I neglected to say, that it was almost hand and glove. They went—as soon as I had those three, that was the end of them and very soon I started the period.

Dr. You know how long you would be out when you had these convulsions? Did the family say how long you'd be unconscious?

Pt. My mother used to say 3 or 4 minutes to up to an hour.

Dr. Besides the convulsions, were there other times that you passed out? Are there any other times that you've ever had any weakness or paralysis or numbness or tingling or anything such as the stroke for even briefly?

Pt. No, no. Other than that, nothing.

Dr. Any pains in your joints or limbs?

Pt. No.

Dr. Any rashes, itching, or skin trouble?

Pt. No.

Return to Family Health. Grandparents.

Dr. How about the health of your grandparents? Do you know anything about their health?

Pt. My grandmother on my father's side was—she was an old lady. And my grandfather on my father's side, he was only 60 and he died of—something wrong with his heart. I don't know what it was. It was so long ago. And my grandfather on my mother's side was just old and my grandmother was—she had a goiter.

Dr. How old was she when she died?

Pt. Oh, I think she was . . . maybe . . . 50, something like that. She wasn't too old.

Dr. And your mother's father you said was how old?

Pt. He was old; 70 . . . almost close to 80.

Dr. And then your grandfather on your father's side was the one who had the heart trouble in his 60's. And his wife?

Pt. She died of old age.

Dr. She was about how old?

Pt. Oh, she was 70 . . . 5, 6.

Dr. Were there any serious illnesses beside what you've mentioned in—say cousins or aunts and uncles, that you know of, any other heart trouble or . . .

Pt. No.

Dr. . . .cancer or birth defects?

Pt. No.

Current living situation.

Dr. One other question occurs to me. You live in a house?

Pt. Mm-hmmm.

Dr. Your own house?

Pt. No.

Dr. Rented?

Pt. Mm-hmmm.

Dr. And what is the house like?

Pt. Well, we live in an apartment upstairs. And it's connected with the Church of Reconciliation. My husband takes care of the church in return for the apartment. We get it rent free and heat and so forth.

Dr. So it's an upstairs apartment?

Pt. Yeah.

Dr. So that means you have to go up a flight of stairs to get to your apartment.

Pt. Hmmmm.

Dr. And how much room do you have?

Pt. Oh, we have six rooms.

Dr. And who's downstairs?

Pt. Nobody.

Interviewer rechecks exertional dyspnea.

Dr. Nobody. Have you noticed any difficulty before you were told not to do much, say in last summer or spring, any problem going upstairs?

Pt. The only time I had trouble going up and down stairs was the early part of the summer. It bothered me to go up and down stairs.

Dr. How?

Pt. By the time I'd get up the stairs, I'd have to sit down in a chair 'cause it would make me so . . . breathe so fast.

Dr. How about your breathing at that time?

Pt. Well, you know, you breathe so fast, so rapid . . . that . . .

Dr. This started when?

Pt. Before I had the first episode in the bank, you know.

Dr. About how long . . . in July or June?

Pt. Yeah.

Dr. And how about carrying your groceries upstairs?

Pt. Well, see, I have a very independent streak (laugh) and I have always done it.

Dr. And did you notice any difficulty with that before then?

Pt. Yeah.

Dr. When did you first notice trouble with carrying groceries up?

Pt. Oh, probably a year before that.

Dr. Have you had to stop doing anything in your housework, such as vacuuming or cleaning the walls or anything like that?

Pt. Yeah.

Dr. When did that start?

Pt. Well, maybe a year before that and so forth.

Patient now acknowledges she was forced to reduce activity 2 years ago.

Dr. Two years ago?

Pt. I think approximately that, I'd say. And then I'd wait until I felt like, you know, just for a few minutes and then I'd go right on.

Dr. You could continue then.

Pt. Yeah.

Dr. It's really been about two years then, hasn't it?

Pt. Yes.

Step 9: Completion of interview

Dr. Well fine, I think I've got a pretty good idea of this illness. Is there anything else you would like to say?

Pt. No, I think that's about all.

The next task is to select from the extensive interview material what information should be recorded and how it should be organized. First, the present illness must be identified. Since the story is consistent with valvular heart disease present for at least 25 years, this entire period should be included in the Present Illness. The neurological illness which occurred 7 weeks before admission should also be included, since the symptoms are recent and are probably related to the patient's heart disease. One begins the Present Illness with a description of the abrupt increase in cardiac symptoms starting in August, 1967, describes the course of the illness up to the time of admission, and follows with the sequence of symptoms as they had developed over the preceding years.

The episode reported as "rheumatic fever" at age eight is only briefly mentioned in Present Illness and is described more fully under Past Health, since it was atypical and not necessarily connected with the current illness. The symptoms of edema and dyspnea associated with the pregnancies are handled in a similar way.

In the Personal and Social History, attention is directed to the patient's personality characteristics, which may have direct bearing on the reliability of the history and the course of the illness. The disturbing events in the patient's recent life are emphasized, particularly her unhappiness over the son's marriage and her unresolved grief consequent to the brother's suicide. The temporal relationship of these two events to the increase in the patient's symptoms may be pertinent to both the course and the prognosis of the current illness.

THE CASE WRITE-UP

VIRGINIA CURTIS
UNIT #52-47-81
FEBRUARY 1, 1968

This is the first Strong Memorial Hospital admission of Mrs. Curtis, a 52-year-old married housewife and bank teller, mother of three, who lives with her husband and two younger children in Geneva, New York. She was admitted January 26, 1968, referred by Drs. Robert Jones and James Watson of Geneva for evaluation of her cardiac status and consideration of cardiac surgery.

SOURCE AND RELIABILITY OF THE HISTORY. The information was obtained from the patient, an intelligent person who tends to minimize symptoms.

PRESENT ILLNESS. The patient has had a history of rapid heart action since 1943 with gradually increasing dyspnea and ankle edema since 1963 or 1964. A diagnosis of rheumatic fever was made at age 8 and a murmur reported at age 27.

On Friday, August 4, 1967, while walking slowly, she suddenly developed severe aching pain in the left anterior upper chest, radiating to the entire left arm, that was associated with dyspnea and a rapid irregular heart beat. With rest, the arm pain subsided in 10 minutes and the chest pain in 20 minutes. Although the rapid heart action persisted, she remained at work for the rest of the afternoon. That evening her physician advised rest over the weekend and prescribed quinidine three times a day. The tachycardia subsided within two days and she returned to work on August 7. The next day she developed malaise, chilly feelings, fever, and sweats, which lasted a few days but were followed by recurrence of tachycardia, dyspnea, and an increase in ankle edema. Unable to perform light household chores, she remained in bed the rest of that week, sleeping with two pillows and occasionally awakening short of breath. She returned to her job on Monday, August 14, but was admitted to the intensive care unit of St. Jerome's Hospital the next day, where she was started on digoxin, a low salt diet, and warfarin. Although her symptoms had improved at discharge on September 3, some tachycardia and dyspnea persisted. Warfarin was discontinued and digoxin was increased to two a day. The consulting cardiologist, Dr. Watson, raised the question of eventual surgical correction and recommended restriction of activities to light housework. Because of no significant improvement over the next 3 months at home, despite restricted activity, the decision was made on November 7, 1967, that she enter Strong Memorial Hospital in January for consideration of cardiac surgery.

On December 11, 1967, she suddenly developed paresthesias of her fingers and weakness of her right hand and arm that rapidly extended to the right face and right leg. She fell when attempting to stand and was unconscious for approximately 10 minutes. Admitted to the intensive care unit of St. Jerome's Hospital, she was confused for 3 or 4 days, paralyzed on the right side, was unable to see to her right, and had difficulty speaking. After a few days, she began to show progressive improvement except for the right arm, which remained paralyzed. During the 5½-week hospital stay the only cardiac symptom was occasional tachycardia. She was discharged on January 17, 1968.

While at home for 9 days awaiting admission to Strong Memorial Hospital, she was markedly fatigued but attempted to resume her usual household activities.

The patient has had a long history of episodes of rapid heart action, the first in 1943 (age 27), 3 months after her first baby died at birth of a "heart ailment," and 6 months after the death of her mother. At that time, she also had "shortness of breath," which was unrelated to exertion, described as a need to sigh. A BMR was normal and she was told she had a "scar in the heart." Thereafter, she periodically noted rapid heart action, particularly in hot weather. During each of her pregnancies (1943, 1946, 1951, and 1957), she had repeated hemoptyses as well as swelling of her legs, which persisted several months after delivery. During the last two pregnancies she also noted exertional dyspnea. Four or 5 years ago (1963 or 1964), mild exertional dyspnea and swelling of the ankles at the end of the day first developed. Two years ago, she began sleeping with two pillows because her "breathing was easier." In June or July, 1966, she had a sudden, marked increase in leg edema, swelling of the abdomen and a gain of 13 pounds, but no increase in dyspnea. An oral diuretic relieved these symptoms in a few days. During the winter of 1966–1967 she had more persistent edema of her legs by evening and intermittent tachycardia. Exertional dyspnea gradually increased so that by the summer of 1967 she had difficulty climbing one flight of stairs, but there was no increase in orthopnea and no paroxysmal nocturnal dyspnea or cough.

Over these 4 to 5 years she has been distressed by family problems, especially the marriage of her son in 1966 and the death by suicide of her youngest brother in March 1967 (see Personal and Social History).

Currently the patient is on a salt-free diet, digitalis, and warfarin (5 mg. daily).

PAST HEALTH

General Health: In spite of the symptoms noted above, the patient considers herself to have been in good health throughout her life.

Childhood Health: Measles and mumps. No scarlet fever or diphtheria.

At age 8 the patient had an illness diagnosed as "rheumatic fever," characterized by painless swelling of both feet and legs, but no pain or swelling of joints, no fever, sore throat, rash, or chorea. There was no known urinary problem or facial edema. She was kept home at rest for a year.

From early childhood to age 14 she had seizures, characterized by her eyes rolling up, followed by loss of consciousness, but no jerking or incontinence.

Age 9, Tonsillectomy.

Adult Health:

MEDICAL ILLNESSES. (See Present Illness.)

SURGICAL PROCEDURES. January 11, 1968, dilatation and curettage for menorrhagia at St. Jerome's Hospital.

PSYCHIATRIC ILLNESSES. None.

OBSTETRICAL HISTORY. 1943 (age 27), first pregnancy: nausea, vomiting, and small hemoptyses throughout the 9 months. The infant died of a "heart ailment" at birth.

1946 (age 30), second pregnancy: nausea, vomiting, epistaxes, occasional small hemoptyses, persistent edema of the legs, and a weight gain of more than 20 pounds. She delivered a full-term, healthy male infant.

1951 (age 35), third pregnancy: nausea, vomiting, hemoptyses, dyspnea, and edema, requiring hospital admission at the third month for intravenous fluids. A healthy male infant was born at term. Dependent edema persisted for 3 months after the delivery.

1957 (age 42), fourth pregnancy: hemorrhage at the second and third months, but she carried the baby, a healthy girl, to term. Again there was nausea, vomiting, edema, hemoptysis, and some dyspnea. This pregnancy was unplanned.

Accidents and Injuries. None.

Allergies. None.

Immunizations. Not asked.

FAMILY HEALTH

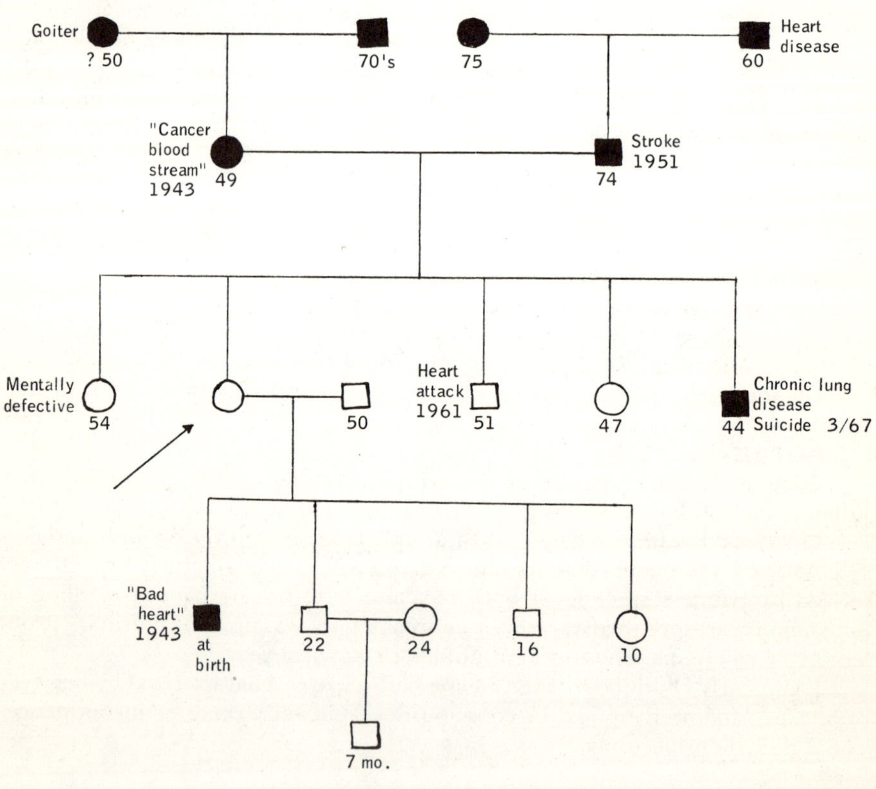

The mother died in 1943, at age 49, during the patient's first pregnancy, with "cancer of the blood," and had been "sickly all the time" with numerous operations. The father had a stroke in March, 1951, and died at home in August, 1951, during the patient's third pregnancy.

Siblings. Bessie, age 54, is living, married, and mentally defective, with two children, one a "Mongolian." John, age 51, had a "heart attack" in 1961, followed by "blood clots." Geraldine, age 47, is in good health except for a hysterectomy a few years ago. Merlin committed suicide by gunshot in March, 1967, age 44. He had chronic lung disease compatible with bronchiectasis, a lobectomy in 1956, and shortly before the suicide a recurrence of pulmonary symptoms.

The patient's three children, Robert, age 22, Mark, 16, Lois, 10, have all been in good health, as has the patient's husband, age 50.

Other than the paternal grandfather and the brother, no one else in the family has had heart disease. There is no family history of cancer, birth defects, or epilepsy. One aunt had a stroke 2 years ago at age 82; she is still living.

PERSONAL AND SOCIAL HISTORY

Current Life Situation. The patient, her husband, and the two younger children occupy a rent-free, six-room apartment on the second floor of a house, in return for which the husband acts as custodian for the church next door. Employed for more than 30 years as a railroad car inspector, he is covered by a company pension and benefits. He works irregular hours, sometimes at night, but he and the children have been able to assist in household chores. The two younger children are in school at appropriate grades. One source of family friction was the engagement and marriage in May, 1966, of the son, Robert, to a girl two years older. The patient opposed the marriage and does not get along with her daughter-in-law, but feels there is nothing further she can do to improve the relationship. She is also still upset about the suicide of Merlin in March, 1967, and did not attend the funeral in Virginia as she feared it would make her sick. She cried when she discussed Merlin's death.

Until August, 1967, the patient had been working for a year as a clerk and bank teller. She has always been a very active, busy person and has found it difficult to be confined to limited activity. Since being ill, she has tried to keep busy by knitting and doing light housework. She needs to present herself as an active, vigorous, and competent person.

Past Development. The patient is the second oldest of five children and was brought up in Geneva, New York, where her father worked as an auto mechanic and truck driver. Because of her mother's chronic ill health and her older sister's mental deficiency, the responsibility for the care of the other children was hers. She finished high school while helping out at home. From 1936 until her first pregnancy in 1943 she worked as a clerk in a paper firm. She married in 1938 but continued to live in the parental home. After her mother's death in 1943, she looked after the mentally deficient sister until she was married and then kept house for her father until his death in 1951, assuming full responsibility for his terminal illness of 6 months.

She is a Protestant and her husband is Catholic.

SYSTEMS REVIEW:[1]

Skin. No rashes or pruritus.

Hematopoietic System. Not asked.

Head and Face. Headaches during pregnancy.

Ears. No difficulty with hearing, tinnitus, or earaches.

Eyes. Glasses for myopia for 20 years; no pain, inflammation, diplopia; visual field defect during stroke (see Present Illness).

Nose and Sinuses. Infrequent colds.

Mouth, Pharynx, and Larynx. A number of teeth have been "abscessed" and extracted. Infrequent sore throats. No dysphagia.

Breasts. Not asked.

Respiratory Tract. No pleurisy. Hemoptysis during pregnancies.

Cardiovascular System. (see Present Illness.)

Gastrointestinal System. Appetite has been good. "Nervous indigestion" as a child. Nausea and vomiting during pregnancies. No jaundice, diarrhea, recent indigestion, or bloody stool. Thrombosed and bleeding hemorrhoids 5 years ago.

Urinary Tract. No history of kidney trouble, back pain, hematuria, nocturia, or enuresis.

Genital Tract. Menarche age 14; last menstrual period, early January 1968. In September 1967, and again in January 1968, she had excessive bleeding.

Skeletal System. No pain in the extremities.

Nervous System. Stroke (see Present Illness). Convulsions (see Past Health).

Endocrine System. In 1943, BMR was normal. Other symptoms not asked.

Psychological Status. (See Personal and Social History.)

PHYSICAL EXAMINATION

RELIABILITY. The patient is cooperative, and the physical examination, done February 1, 1968, is complete.

GENERAL DESCRIPTION. Mrs. Curtis is slight of build, wears glasses, and has graying hair. There is slight hirsutism, including hair on the upper lip and a small amount on her lateral chin. She appears calm, is cheerful, responsive, cooperative, and tries to do things for herself. She is well oriented. Her speech is occasionally hesitant with slight evidence of an expressive aphasia, but she is able to speak her words distinctly. She rises easily from her chair to walk down the corridor without any trace of a limp. There is little motion of her right arm as she walks, and during the examination she frequently holds her right hand with her left.

VITAL SIGNS. Blood pressure 100/62 mm. Hg (recumbent) in both arms. Radial pulse totally irregular at 88 beats/min.; with 10 sit-ups rises to 104. Apical rate 96 beats/min. Respirations normal.

---

[1] The Systems Review is not complete. Those symptoms not inquired about during the first interview, as well as other omissions in the history, would normally be pursued in a subsequent patient visit before writing the case history.

SKIN. Normal color, a few small angiomata on the anterior chest; an irregular pale 2 × 4 cm. flat, pink hemangioma on the middle of the upper left anterior thigh, and also a similar lesion is present on the midlateral anterior left calf, measuring 4 × 6 cm. There is an old scar 4 cm. long below the right knee cap (from a fall in childhood), and two or three fresh scratch marks on both upper lateral forearms caused by her pet cat.

LYMPHATIC SYSTEM. Two discrete, soft, 1 cm. right posterior cervical nodes; no other nodes felt.

SKULL. Normal.

FACE. Slight flattening of right nasolabial fold. (See neurological examination.)

EYES. Patient reads 2 mm. print with bifocals at 2 feet. Sclerae and conjunctivae normal. Pupils equal, 4 mm., react to light and accommodation. Extraocular motions normal. Visual fields are full. Right fundus is at −1; left at 0 diopters. Disc margins are sharp. Normal arterioles and veins with no nicking. No hemorrhages or exudates. Maculae normal.

EARS. Whispered voice is heard equally well in both ears without difficulty. The right canal is occluded with cerumen; the left canal, narrow. Only the anterior part of the left tympanic membrane is seen, which is of normal color.

NOSE. No lesions, septum slightly deviated to the left but with normal patency.

TEETH. Gums in good repair. No lesions. Two premolars missing in the right lower jaw; third molars missing on each side of the lower jaw. Teeth filled with amalgam fillings.

PHARYNX. Not inflamed. No tonsils seen. Tongue coated.

NECK. Left lobe of thyroid is palpable, not visible, normal in size. Isthmus not felt. No pyramidal lobe.

BREASTS. Only a small amount of glandular tissue with no masses. Nipples prominent, no abnormalities.

THORAX AND LUNGS. Slight scoliosis of the middorsal spine to the left; equal expansion of each hemithorax. Breath sounds are normal. Normal tactile and vocal fremitus. Normal percussion. Diaphragms move equally 3 cm. bilaterally. No rales or wheezes.

CARDIOVASCULAR SYSTEM

Heart. No abnormal pulsations are seen. There is no right ventricular lift. The apical impulse is discrete with a very slight localized thrust 11 cm. to the left of the midsternal line in the fifth intercostal space. The intensity of the first heart sound at the apex is slightly increased and sharp. There is also a slight increase in intensity of the second sound heard in the pulmonic area, which is greater than a normal second sound in the aortic area. There is an opening snap moderately close to the second sound, heard best to the left of the low sternum. No splitting. No basilar murmurs. No left sternal border diastolic murmur. There is a grade 2/6 blowing apical systolic murmur going two-thirds of the way through systole that dies out in the midaxillary line and is also heard to the left of the low sternum. In left lateral position there is a grade 2/6 rumbling diastolic murmur, which occupies all of diastole when the ventricular rate is slow. No gallop.

Peripheral Vascular. No jugular venous distention at 45 degrees. No abnormal venous pulsations. Carotid arteries show normal pulsations of equal intensity, and there are no bruits. The abdominal aorta is normal, easily felt, and measures 3½ cm. in breadth. There is a faint late systolic bruit heard above the umbilicus, that fades out toward the upper abdomen. The peripheral pulses (0-4+) are as follows:

	CAROTID	RADIAL	FEMORAL	POPLITEAL	DORSALIS PEDIS	POSTERIOR TIBIAL
right	+++	+++	+++	+++	+++	+
left	+++	+++	+++	+++	+++	?

There is no pretibial or sacral edema.

ABDOMEN. Scaphoid. No abnormal pulsations or masses. Active peristalsis is heard and is of normal pitch. The liver edge just descends to the costal margin on deep inspiration and is nontender. The span of total liver dullness measures 10 cm. The spleen is not palpable. The lower pole of the right kidney is just felt; the lower pole of the left kidney is not felt. The sigmoid colon is palpable as a soft, cylindrical structure.

GENITAL EXAMINATION. Normal female escutcheon. Labia, urethral meatus, and vaginal introitus appear normal. There is no tenderness and no discharge. The cervix looks normal and is firm, freely movable, and nontender. The uterus is small, firm, without irregularities, and nontender. The ovaries are not palpable. No masses or tenderness in the cul-de-sac.

RECTAL EXAMINATION. Normal sphincter tone. No pain or tenderness. No masses. Brownish stool on examining finger, guaiac negative.

SKELETAL SYSTEM. Normal.

NEUROLOGICAL EXAMINATION

General Status. See above for general description.

Cranial Nerves. I - not tested; II - normal (see above); III, IV, VI - normal (see above); V - normal light touch and pain sensation to pin prick, equal bilaterally; corneal reflexes are equal. Motor V - normal with patient biting down. VII - slight flattening of right nasolabial fold. Symmetrical smile; patient able to wrinkle forehead bilaterally. VIII - gross testing normal. IX, X - uvula moves in midline; slight gag reflex, equal bilaterally. XI - weakness in sternocleidomastoids bilaterally. Slight decrease of strength in right shoulder with elevation. XII - tongue in midline with good force in both cheeks.

Motor System. No abnormality in the strength of the left arm or two lower extremities. Normal gait. The patient is able to rise from a squatting position or from a chair without difficulty, and can stand on toes and heels. The right arm is considerably weak, more so proximally; she can make a fist, but grasp is weak. She can extend and flex wrist against gravity, but there is considerable weakness. Pronation and supination of the forearm are done weakly but can be done against gravity. Twenty per cent limitation of full supination. Full range of motion at elbow, which is able to move against gravity. Marked weakness of the shoulder in all directions. No pain. No fasciculation or atrophy. The skin of the fingers of right hand is slightly shiny, and there is minimal edema.

Coordination: Finger-to-nose on the left is normal and cannot be done on the right. Heel-to-shin bilaterally normal. In putting on her gown, she uses mainly the left arm but is able to lift the right arm enough to direct it into the sleeve. Romberg's test is negative.

Sensory System. Response to light touch, pin prick, position, and vibration is normal and equal bilaterally. Two point sense is intact on hand and forearm, and there is no extinction phenomenon.

Reflexes. Note that the right deep tendon reflexes are more active than the left and that the plantar responses are flexor.

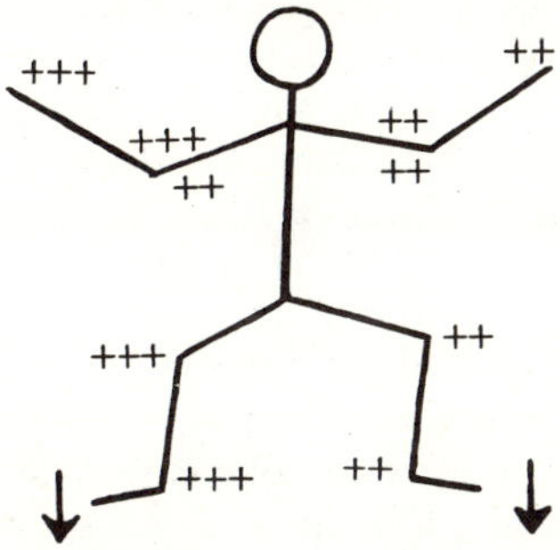

Spinal Nerve Irritation. Negative.

DIAGNOSIS

The patient, who is 52 years old with possible rheumatic fever at age 8, has had an intermittent cardiac irregularity for 25 years and the gradual progression of dyspnea, orthopnea, and dependent edema over 4 to 5 years. She was hospitalized in August, 1967, for the sudden onset of cardiac irregularity, chest pain, and increased dyspnea. Since then she has been digitalized, placed on a low salt diet, and her activity restricted, without improvement. On December 11, 1967, she was hospitalized with a right hemiplegia of sudden onset, which cleared over 5½ weeks except for weakness of the right arm. She is referred for the consideration of cardiac surgery. On physical examination there is a totally irregular pulse, a grade 2/6 apical systolic murmur, a full length grade 2/6 mitral diastolic rumble, and an opening snap. There are no signs of neck vein distention, pulmonary congestion, or edema. The right arm and face are weak and there is hyperreflexia on the right.

The cardiac findings are classically those of mitral stenosis and mitral regurgitation, the predominant lesion being mitral stenosis. The full length diastolic rumble at a slow ventricular rate means that there is a continuous pressure gradient between the left atrium and left ventricle throughout diastole, that the left atrium cannot empty completely, and consequently the degree of stenosis is severe. The loud mitral first heart sound and opening snap suggest that the valve, though scarred, is still flexible and that mitral stenosis predominates. If there were a severe degree of mitral regurgitation causing valve destruction and allowing rapid ventricular filling, the opening snap would be absent and the intensity of the first mitral sound decreased. The grade 2 mitral systolic murmur, which is not holosystolic, probably represents a minimal degree of mitral regurgitation. Tricuspid regurgitation is an alternative diagnosis since the systolic murmur was also heard at the sternum, but there is no accentuated *v* wave in the jugular venous pulse and the murmur is also transmitted to the axilla. The history of a "scar" in the heart 25 years ago supports the diagnosis of rheumatic heart disease, although the illness at age 8 is atypical in that the swelling of the legs is reported as painless.

The history of periodic irregular heart action since 1945 is compatible with paroxysmal atrial fibrillation, which is not uncommon in mitral stenosis, but these symptoms could also have been due to intermittent premature beats. The possibility of thyrotoxicosis might be considered, even though the patient volunteers no symptoms of hyperthyroidism, the thyroid gland is not enlarged, and the BMR was normal when palpitations first appeared.

The symptoms of congestive heart failure began 4 or 5 years ago, but may also have been present during the three pregnancies in 1946, 1951, and 1957, precipitated by the increased blood volume of pregnancy. Hemoptysis is not uncommon in the early stages of mitral stenosis resulting from increased pulmonary venous pressure and rupture of pulmonary veins at the time that pulmonary arteriolar resistance is low. Since the edema seemed to be out of proportion to the dyspnea and persisted several months postpartum, one would also have to consider other causes for the edema. Deep leg vein thrombosis would be a possibility; however, the lack of pain, recurrence with each pregnancy, and symmetrical distribution of edema would be against the diagnosis. Edema at age 8 suggests renal disease, but other findings such as hypertension, progressive difficulty with each pregnancy, and urinary findings of residual renal disease are absent.

The gradually developing dyspnea, orthopnea, and more persistent ankle edema 4 to 5 years ago marks the beginning of cardiac decompensation. The sighing type of respiration in 1943 that occurred soon after the death of the patient's mother and infant son "with a heart ailment" is clearly not cardiac dyspnea and more likely represents a conversion symptom.

The episode of cardiac irregularity and transient pain in August, 1967, suggests the sudden onset of atrial fibrillation with a rapid ventricular rate resulting in decreased cardiac output and coronary insufficiency. The patient has continued in atrial fibrillation since August. The absence of effective left atrial contraction and consequent impairment of left ventricular filling as a result of atrial fibrillation, coupled with tight mitral stenosis, has led to a decrease in cardiac output and more congestive heart failure. The psychologic strain of the past 4 or 5 years, to which she has responded by becoming more active and by denying disability, may have led the patient to ignore warning signals and to exert herself beyond her cardiac reserve.

The sudden right hemiparesis, aphasia, and right homonymous hemianopsia of December 11, 1967, suggest an arterial obstruction in the distribution of the left middle cerebral artery. The pyramidal system, the expressive speech areas of the temporal lobe, and the optic radiation were all involved. The abrupt onset without premonitory signs and the relatively rapid improvement in spite of massive involvement is typical of a cerebral embolus. One may postulate vasospasm involving the vascular tree distal to the point of impact and then recovery of function as the spasm relaxed and the embolus moved forward to a smaller vessel. Such a course is unusual with cerebral thrombosis or cerebral hemorrhage. Embolization is common with mitral stenosis and atrial fibrillation where there is stasis of blood in the left atrium and formation of clot. There are no symptoms or signs to invoke the diagnosis of bacterial endocarditis as a cause for the embolism; the history of possible rheumatic fever, as well as the scarred valve 25 years ago, rules against the rare left atrial myxoma, which also is a cause of systemic embolism.

DIAGNOSES

1. Chronic rheumatic heart disease with predominant mitral stenosis and slight mitral regurgitation, Functional Class III.
2. Atrial fibrillation.
3. Congestive heart failure (by history).
4. Right arm paresis, secondary to left middle cerebral artery embolus (6 weeks ago).
5. Depression, occult.

PROGNOSIS

The evidence of slowly developing cardiac decompensation over a 4 or 5 year period with progression over the past 5 months, despite considerable restriction of activity, a low-salt diet, and digitalization, speaks for a very guarded prognosis. Persistent atrial fibrillation and an episode of cerebral embolization with residual neurological deficits also limit the outlook. The problem is further compounded by the patient's proclivity to deny symptoms, which may mean that the degree of failure is even greater than she has reported. On the surface, she seems cheerful enough, but underneath there is evidence of a significant depression, related to the brother's suicide, and also, no doubt, to the consequence of having to restrict her activity because of illness.

If further studies support the impression that the patient has tight mitral stenosis and minimal mitral regurgitation, she should be a reasonable risk for mitral commissurotomy. The recent evidence for clot in the left atrium would favor a commissurotomy done under direct vision, with cardiac bypass rather than a closed procedure, even though the latter operation carries a slightly higher risk. Without surgery, the patient's prognosis is one of a progressively downhill course. Knowing the importance for this woman to be active, one would predict that she would be in favor of commissurotomy. There is no evidence that she exploits symptoms or has accepted chronic illness as a way of life which she would be reluctant to abandon. Hence, any measure which would enhance her range of activity would also be expected to have a favorable psychological impact.

Index